Surgery of Shoulder Instability

W0050045

Surface Science Techniques

Stephen F. Brockmeier
Mark D. Miller · Guillermo Arce

Editors

Surgery of Shoulder Instability

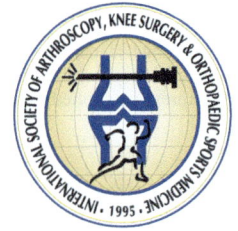

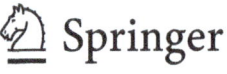

Editors
Stephen F. Brockmeier
Department of Orthopaedic Surgery
University of Virginia
Charlottesville, VA
USA

Mark D. Miller
Department of Orthopaedic Surgery
University of Virginia
Charlottesville, VA
USA

Guillermo Arce
Department of Orthopaedic Surgery
Instituto Argentino de Diagnóstico
  y Tratamiento
Buenos Aires
Argentina

ISBN 978-3-642-38099-0   ISBN 978-3-642-38100-3   (eBook)
DOI 10.1007/978-3-642-38100-3
Springer Heidelberg New York Dordrecht London

Library of Congress Control Number: 2013937198

© ISAKOS 2013
This work is subject to copyright. All rights are reserved by the Publisher, whether the whole or part of the material is concerned, specifically the rights of translation, reprinting, reuse of illustrations, recitation, broadcasting, reproduction on microfilms or in any other physical way, and transmission or information storage and retrieval, electronic adaptation, computer software, or by similar or dissimilar methodology now known or hereafter developed. Exempted from this legal reservation are brief excerpts in connection with reviews or scholarly analysis or material supplied specifically for the purpose of being entered and executed on a computer system, for exclusive use by the purchaser of the work. Duplication of this publication or parts thereof is permitted only under the provisions of the Copyright Law of the Publisher's location, in its current version, and permission for use must always be obtained from Springer. Permissions for use may be obtained through RightsLink at the Copyright Clearance Center. Violations are liable to prosecution under the respective Copyright Law. The use of general descriptive names, registered names, trademarks, service marks, etc. in this publication does not imply, even in the absence of a specific statement, that such names are exempt from the relevant protective laws and regulations and therefore free for general use.
While the advice and information in this book are believed to be true and accurate at the date of publication, neither the authors nor the editors nor the publisher can accept any legal responsibility for any errors or omissions that may be made. The publisher makes no warranty, express or implied, with respect to the material contained herein.

Printed on acid-free paper

Springer is part of Springer Science+Business Media (www.springer.com)

Preface

On behalf of the International Society of Arthroscopy, Knee Surgery, and Orthopedic Sports Medicine (ISAKOS), we are proud to introduce one of the first of what we hope will be a long-standing and successful venture ISAKOS topical booklets. This booklet on Shoulder Instability truly lives up to this concept, it is international in every sense of the word, and it provides a state-of-the-art update on this topic. We are excited that ISAKOS has partnered with Springer publishing to produce these topical booklets, and are honored that we were given the opportunity to participate.

This booklet covers the entire gambit of surgical management of shoulder instability—from the first time dislocator to the management of complex chronic cases. The author list is a virtual Who's Who among international shoulder surgeons. No shoulder surgeon should be without this important work.

Again, we emphasize that this booklet is a stand-alone treatise on this important sports medicine topic. Much appreciation to ISAKOS, Springer, and Dr. Stephen Brockmeier, who was the lead editor on this topic. We look forward to many more successful topical booklets in the future.

Mark D. Miller MD

Contents

Acute Traumatic Anterior Shoulder Instability: Surgical Management for the First-Time Dislocator

1

Patrick N. Siparsky and Dean C. Taylor

1.1 Introduction

The complex relationship between increased range of motion and decreased stability subjects the shoulder to more episodes of subluxation and dislocation than other joints in the body. Traumatic anterior glenohumeral dislocation remains a common problem not only in young athletes, but also for older individuals after a fall. The most common mechanism of injury remains shoulder abduction with forced external rotation that often results in significant disability and time lost from work or sports.

1.1.1 Static and Dynamic Stabilizers of the Glenohumeral Joint

The shoulder is a complex joint composed of static and dynamic stabilizers. (Table 1.1) The stability of the shoulder is dependent on the structural and functional relationships between these components. The static restraints to glenohumeral motion include the normal version and articular surface congruity of the joint, the negative intra-articular pressure of the joint, the glenohumeral ligaments, and the labrum. There is significant variability in the "normal" version of the proximal humerus as was shown by Boileau and Walsh [1]; however, a proximal humerus retroversion angle of approximately 20° compared to the transepicondylar axis of

Disclosure Statement: The authors of this manuscript have no financial disclosures related to this scholarly work, and have received no financial reimbursement for this work. There was no internal or external funding for this work.

P. N. Siparsky (✉) · D. C. Taylor
Duke Sports Medicine Center, Duke University Medical Center, Box 3615, NC 27710, Durham, U.K
e-mail: patrick.siparsky@duke.edu

S. F. Brockmeier et al. (eds.), *Surgery of Shoulder Instability*, DOI: 10.1007/978-3-642-38100-3_1, © ISAKOS 2013

Table 1.1 Static and dynamic stabilizers of the glenohumeral joint

Static Stabilizers	Dynamic Stabilizers
Normal glenoid and humeral version	Rotator cuff muscles
Negative intra-articular pressure	Tendon of the long head of the biceps
The glenohumeral ligaments	Periscapular muscles
Labrum	

the distal humerus was average amongst a large cadaveric study group. The glenoid version is also variable, but typically displays a few degrees of retroversion in the plane of the scapula [2]. Despite the protective nature of the retroversion built into the bony anatomy of the glenohumeral joint, anterior dislocation remains the most common direction of injury.

The glenohumeral ligaments are static restraints to glenohumeral motion dependent on different degrees of flexion/extension and rotation. For example, the superior glenohumeral ligament prevents inferior translation of the humeral head with the arm in the neutral position while the middle glenohumeral ligament prevents anterior translation with the arm in approximately 45° abduction and external rotation [3]. The glenoid labrum is responsible for deepening the articulation between the glenoid and the humeral head, which helps to maintain the negative intra-articular pressure of the shoulder joint. The labrum also serves as the site of attachment for the inferior glenohumeral ligament complex (anterior/inferior) and the biceps tendon (superior).

The dynamic stabilizers of the glenohumeral joint are the rotator cuff muscles, the biceps tendon, and the periscapular muscles. The rotator cuff is critical to the normal biomechanics of the shoulder joint. The main function of these muscles is to compress the humeral head into the glenoid, while also providing a depressive force on the humeral head within the glenoid. This maximizes the lever arm of the deltoid, while providing stability within the shoulder joint. The long head of the biceps tendon also serves to depress the humeral head. The periscapular muscles are critical for stabilization of the glenohumeral joint as they help control the position of the glenoid (part of the scapula) relative to the humeral head.

1.1.2 Pathology of the Traumatic First-Time Dislocation

Traumatic shoulder dislocations can occur via many different mechanisms ranging from sport activities to motor vehicle and bicycle accidents. The most common direction of traumatic glenohumeral dislocation remains anterior. During an episode of shoulder abduction and forced external rotation, the humeral head places significant stress on the anterior inferior labrum. At the time of dislocation, the humeral head experiences axial loading, external rotation, and anterior translation. The pathoanatomy of the traumatic anterior dislocation in young patients is typically the Bankart lesion (also known as the Perthes-Bankart lesion), where the anterior-inferior capsulolabral complex is forcefully pulled from the glenoid during the dislocation [4, 5]. With the capsulolabral complex stripped from the glenoid, the humeral head is no longer stabilized by the deepening effect of the labrum. This injury can also present with a bony fragment attached to the cap-sulolabral complex resulting in additional instability due to decreased glenohu-meral articulation. The greater the axial load, the higher the likelihood of a large glenoid bone defect occurring [6].

In addition to glenoid and labral damage, an impaction fracture on the postero-lateral aspect of the humeral head is commonly present. Often referred to as the Hill-Sachs lesion, this defect results from the humeral head being forcefully externally rotated in abduction until the posterolateral aspect of the humeral head hits the glenoid [7]. A sizeable defect can complicate treatment if the shoulder arc of motion is interrupted by engagement of the humeral head defect on the glenoid articulation.

While approximately 80 % of traumatic anterior glenohumeral dislocations result in soft tissue or bony Bankart lesions, several other soft tissue injuries can lead to recurrent instability. When the Bankart lesion is not the offending pathologic entity, the typical injury occurs to the capsule or capsular attachments to the labrum or humerus. These injuries include the humeral avulsion of the glenohumeral lig-aments (HAGL), the reverse HAGL (RHAGL), the bony HAGL (BHAGL), and the glenoid avulsion of the glenohumeral ligaments (GAGL) [8–10]. The HAGL may be responsible for between 7 and 9 % of all anterior glenohumeral instability [9, 11]. Each of these injuries can contribute to anterior instability and every effort must be made by the clinician to recognize them.

1.1.3   Learning from Long-Term Follow-up of Traumatic Shoulder Dislocations

Arguably, the greatest challenge of dealing with first-time traumatic anterior instability is deciding which patients may benefit from surgical intervention. Despite the lack of consensus regarding exact recurrence rates, many authors agree that younger (age < 25) males have the highest recurrence rates when treated non-operatively [12–27]. This population is also most likely to suffer a traumatic anterior dislocation. Recurrence rates in this population can approach 100 %.

While the high rate of recurrence was previously thought to be isolated to military personnel and high-level contact athletes due to the nature of work or sport, it is now clear that all young males bear the risk of recurrent injury after initial traumatic dislocation. For males less than 25-years old treated non-opera-tively, Robinson et al. reported a 77 % chance of recurrent dislocation for athletes and 81 % for non-athletes at two years. By five years post-dislocation, both groups had an 85 % chance of recurrent instability [24]. It is also clear that there is more to successful treatment of instability than simply avoiding recurrence. Sachs et al. showed that patients who cope with instability (and do not achieve early stability) have lower functional outcome scores than those who undergo surgical stabil-ization of their Bankart lesion [25]. This benefit spread across multiple different scoring systems including the American Shoulder and Elbow Society scale

(ASES), Constant- Murley scale, and the Western Ontario Shoulder Instability Index (WOSI) scores. This outcome suggests that while avoidance of recurrence is imperative, each patient's ability to deal with work, sport, social, lifestyle, and emotional aspects of the injury also factor into successful recovery.

As the body of evidence-based literature regarding traumatic anterior shoulder instability grows, models are being created to provide outcome information for operative versus non-operative treatment for patients of varying ages, activity levels, etc. The value of this modeling is that it can apply subjective patient-derived factors with objective functional data to stratify treatment options. Mather et al. [18] designed a Decision Analysis Model that used the validated WOSI [28] score as the primary outcome measure, with secondary measures including risk of one year and overall instability, stability at 10 years, risk of future surgery, and risk of revision surgery. All of the data that created these models were from level I or II studies only. [12–15, 17, 22, 23].

In the future, this will be a publically available tool for patients and physicians to become more informed regarding potential surgical outcomes based on individual information. Using a computer program, the physician can enter information into the model to help assess factors such as rate of recurrent dislocation. For example, the Decision Analysis Model shows that an 18-year old male treated non-operatively has a 77 % risk of recurrent dislocation within the first year and only a 32 % chance of having a stable shoulder at 10 years. When treated operatively, the recurrence rate is only 17 %. Conversely, a 30-year old female painter (significant overhead activity) also treated non-operatively has a 34 % chance of recurrent instability at one year and a 62 % chance of having a stable shoulder at 10 years [18]. Her recurrence rate if treated operatively with early arthroscopic labral repair is 23 %. This modeling system provides personalized patient care, allowing various factors to help make the best decision for each patient.

1.2   History and Clinical Exam

Acute traumatic dislocations are rarely subtle in nature. The patient will usually recall a significant event and the onset of immediate pain. It can be helpful to understand the exact mechanism of injury, specifically the position of the arm with respect to abduction and rotation, as well as contact or a non-contact injury pattern [19]. When the shoulder is dislocated anteriorly, the arm is often held by the contralateral hand in a position of internal rotation or with the arm folded across the belly. There may be a bulge over the anterior inferior aspect of the shoulder. Even if the diagnosis of dislocation is clear, a neurovascular exam is necessary prior to reduction. At a minimum, the sensory and motor function at the hand (radial, median, and ulnar nerves), elbow flexion strength (musculocutaneous nerve), and sensory function over the lateral aspect of the upper arm (axillary nerve) should be fully tested.

At the time of injury or initial evaluation, it is helpful to discuss any past shoulder injuries or operations. Should the patient describe prior history of laxity, the examining physician must establish whether this laxity (asymptomatic hypermobility of the joint) results in symptomatic instability (abnormal translation leading to symptoms). An exam of the contralateral shoulder should be part of the routine evaluation of any shoulder dislocation.

Once the shoulder is reduced, or if the patient comes to the office with the shoulder already reduced, it is important to perform another neurovascular exam. Determine if any axillary nerve injury has occurred by testing both deltoid sensory and motor function. Between 20 and 50 % of patients sustaining a traumatic anterior dislocation will experience some type of neurologic deficit, though this is often neuropraxia and will resolve [29]. Documentation of a thorough neurologic exam is critical, and discussion with the patient regarding expectations may help in the recovery process.

Once the shoulder has been relocated, there are several specific tests for instability that should be completed to help evaluate each patient that has sustained a traumatic shoulder dislocation. While the focus of this testing is clearly directed at stability, the physician should evaluate the entirety of shoulder function to rule out any other associated injuries. These tests focus on evaluating range of motion, strength, and stability. Strength and range of motion of both shoulders should be assessed to confirm that no injury to the rotator cuff has occurred. In any patient over 40 years of age with a shoulder dislocation, a rotator cuff tear should be presumed until proven otherwise by exam, MRI or both (Fig. 1.1).

The sulcus sign, apprehension test, relocation test, surprise test, and the load-and-shift tests are all helpful in assessing shoulder laxity. The sulcus sign is performed by simply applying longitudinal traction to the arm while it rests at the patient's side [19, 30]. We stabilize the humeral head in the anterior-posterior direction while applying longitudinal traction in order to avoid confusion between inferior translation of the humeral head and anterior-inferior subluxation

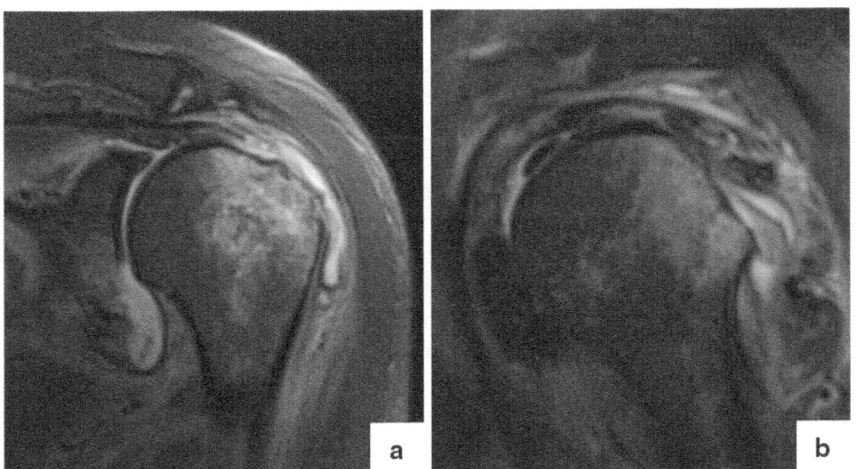

Fig. 1.1 71-year old male after left shoulder dislocation. **a/b** T2 coronal (**a**) and sagittal (**b**) MRI showing associated rotator cuff tear after dislocation (*Images courtesy* of Dr. Grant Garrigues)

Fig. 1.2 Sulcus sign. Inferior translational force is applied to the humerus with the patient in seated position or standing. The humeral head is held in neutral alignment with the glenoid to avoid confusing inferior translation with anterior-inferior subluxation. Grading is based on distance between humeral head and lateral inferior border of acromion

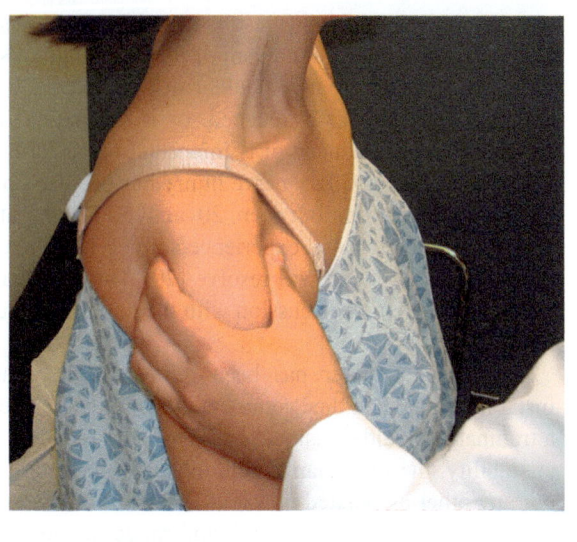

(Fig. 1.2). The test is measured as any displacement of the humeral head from the inferior aspect of the acromion.

The (anterior) apprehension, relocation, and surprise tests are a colection of tests done together to assess anterior glenohumeral stability (Fig. 1.3). These tests are best done with the patient in the supine position and the shoulder in a position of abduction and external rotation. With progressive external rotation, the patient feels a sense of apprehension as the humeral head begins to subluxate over the anterior rim of the glenoid (anterior apprehension test) (Fig. 1.3a). The relocation test counters this maneuver by applying a posteriorly directed force from the examiner's hand directly over the humeral head. This relocation force should alleviate the patient's sense of apprehension and should also allow additional external rotation without pain (Fig. 1.3b). The surprise test is removal of the posteriorly directed force from the relocation maneuver resulting in reproduction of the patient's symptoms as the humeral head translates anteriorly without the opposing force (Fig. 1.3c) [31].

Finally, the load-and-shift test assesses laxity of the glenohumeral joint in various directions and helps delineate the location of the soft tissue lesion (Fig. 1.4). In the clinical setting, this test looks for reproduction of symptoms based on forced translation as described below. In the operating room with the patient relaxed, this test assesses laxity through the amount of humeral head translation on the glenoid. This test is done with one hand on the patient's elbow, applying an axial load to center the humeral head on the glenoid. Then anterior, posterior, and inferior forces are applied separately at varying degrees of shoulder abduction. Typically, this test is done at 0°, 45°, and 90° of abduction. With progressively increasing shoulder abduction, a positive test indicates superior, middle, and inferior glenohumeral ligament laxity or injury. The translation can be graded as well. Grade 1 indicates any humeral head translation to the glenoid rim. Grade 2 indicates humeral head translation over the glenoid rim, but with

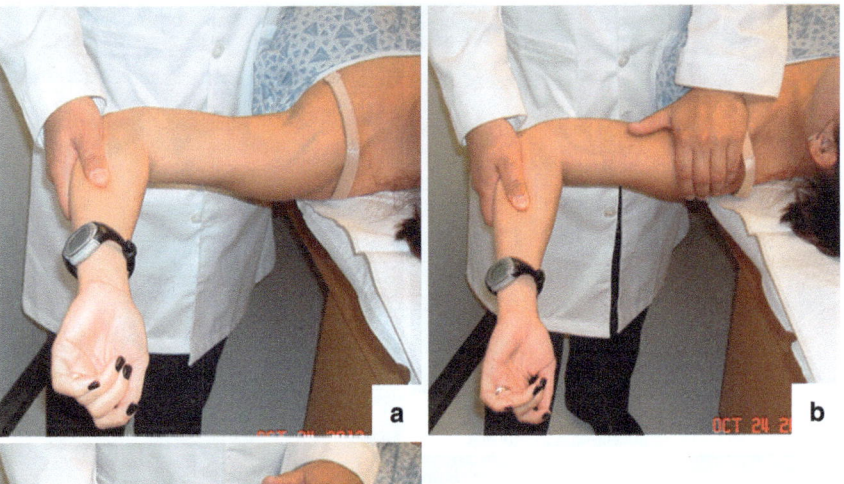

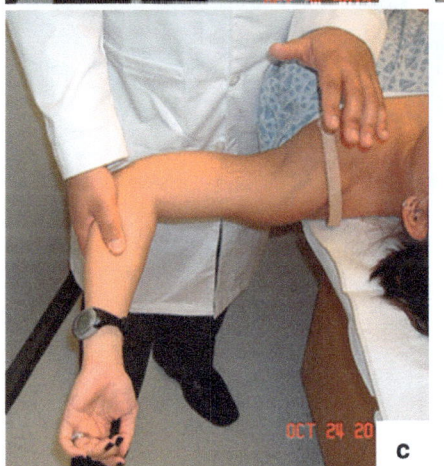

Fig. 1.3 Apprehension-Relocation-Surprise testing for anterior shoulder instability. **a** The patient in the supine position with shoulder abducted and externally rotated to 90°, reporting sensation of anterior instability with continued external rotation. **b** Posterior force applied with palm of examiner's hand relieves sensation of anterior instability. To be positive, further external rotation should be accomplished with no increased apprehension. **c** With removal of the posterior force from the examiner's hand, the patient gets immediate sense of recurrent apprehension as anterior translation of the humeral head recurs

spontaneous reduction. Grade 3 indicates humeral head translation over the glenoid rim that does not spontaneously reduce.

1.3 Imaging

Plain radiographs are used for the initial stages of treatment after dislocation. Anterior-posterior (AP), axillary lateral, and scapular Y views are routinely ordered. The West Point axillary view is also useful in identifying any anterior

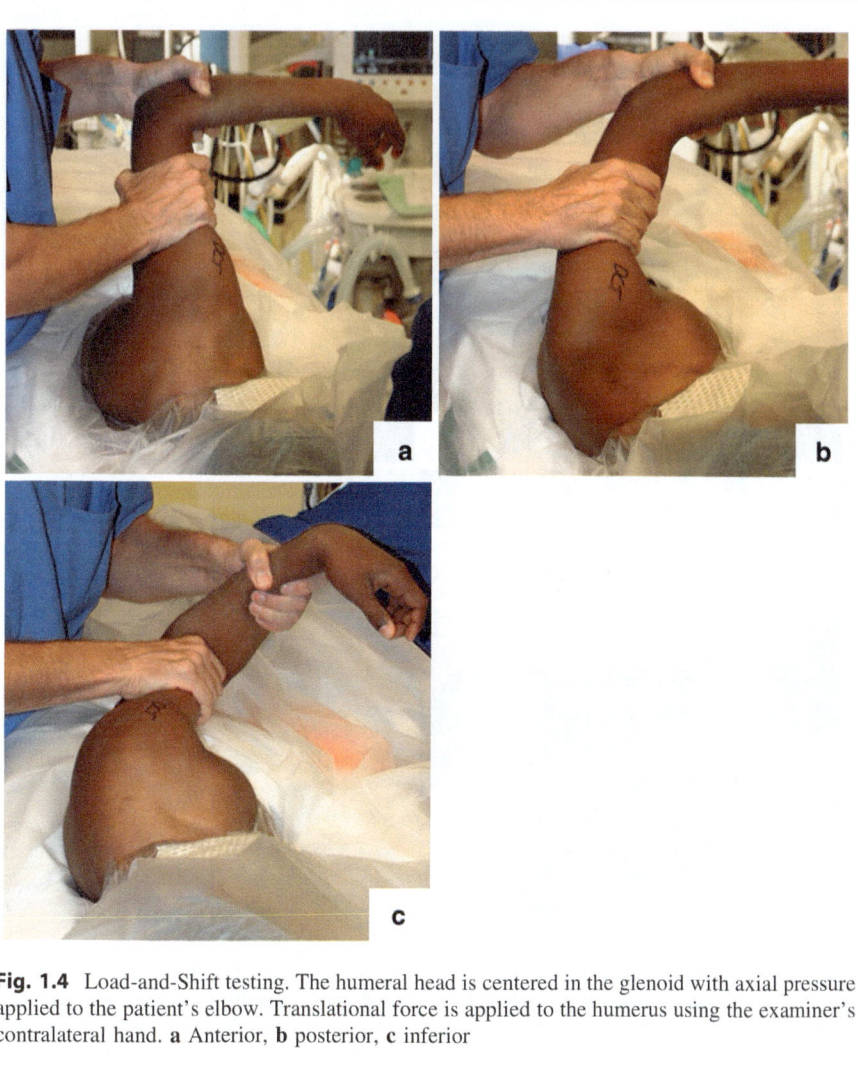

Fig. 1.4 Load-and-Shift testing. The humeral head is centered in the glenoid with axial pressure applied to the patient's elbow. Translational force is applied to the humerus using the examiner's contralateral hand. **a** Anterior, **b** posterior, **c** inferior

inferior glenoid abnormalities (Fig. 1.5). Position the patient prone on the X-ray table with a pillow under the affected shoulder. The shoulder is lifted approximately 8 cm off the table, and the elbow is flexed to 90° and hung off the edge of the table. The X-ray cassette is positioned on the superior aspect of the shoulder and the X-ray beam is then aimed 25° to the patient's midline and 25° to the table surface [32].

It is important to determine the presence of any of the following bony abnormalities while looking at the plain radiographs: Hill-Sachs lesion, greater tuberosity fracture, and anterior inferior glenoid avulsion type fracture (bony Bankart lesion). An MRI helps to visualize any further soft tissue injury. While hemarthrosis may provide an adequate early contrast for looking at labral injury on MRI,

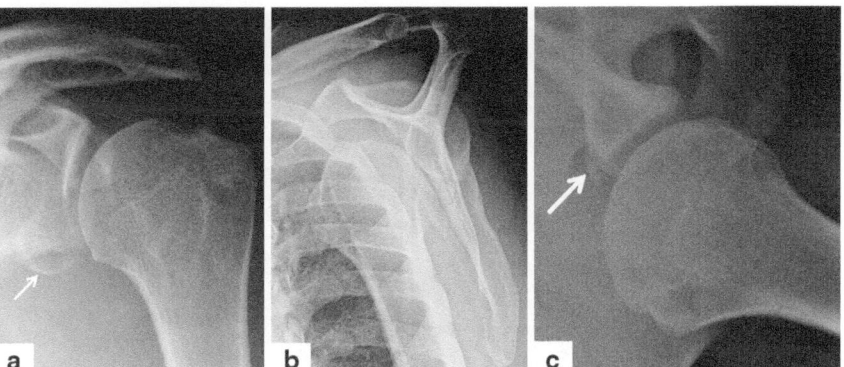

Fig. 1.5 Radiograph series of several different patients. **a** Left AP shoulder X-ray with large Bankart fragment (*arrow*). **b** Scapular Y of dislocated left shoulder. **c** West point axillary X-ray showing glenoid rim fracture (*arrow*) (*Images courtesy* of Dr. Grant Garrigues)

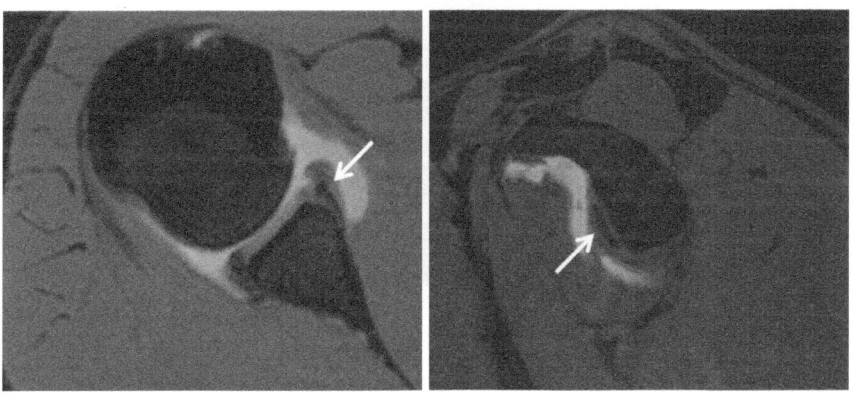

Fig. 1.6 MRI arthrogram of traumatic anterior instability. **a** Axial, **b** sagittal cuts showing large anterior bony Bankart with capsulolabral attachment (*arrows*)

an arthrogram can assist in defining any labral injuries (Fig. 1.6). In the absence of a clear Bankart lesion, suspect the presence of an injury to one of the glenohumeral ligaments, specifically the humeral avulsion of the glenohumeral ligaments (HAGL) lesion (Fig. 1.7).

A CT scan should be reserved for evaluation of significant glenoid bone loss. 3-D reconstructions can be helpful in defining the exact location and shape of the bone loss (Fig. 1.8). With greater than 25 % bone loss, it is unlikely that an arthroscopic Bankart repair will be able to restore glenohumeral stability. The CT scan can help determine the amount of bone necessary for sufficient restoration of glenohumeral stability, whether this is from a Laterjet procedure (corocoid), iliac crest bone graft (autograft), or distal tibial allograft [33]. Each of these techniques can help provide bony stability in the presence of significant glenoid bone loss.

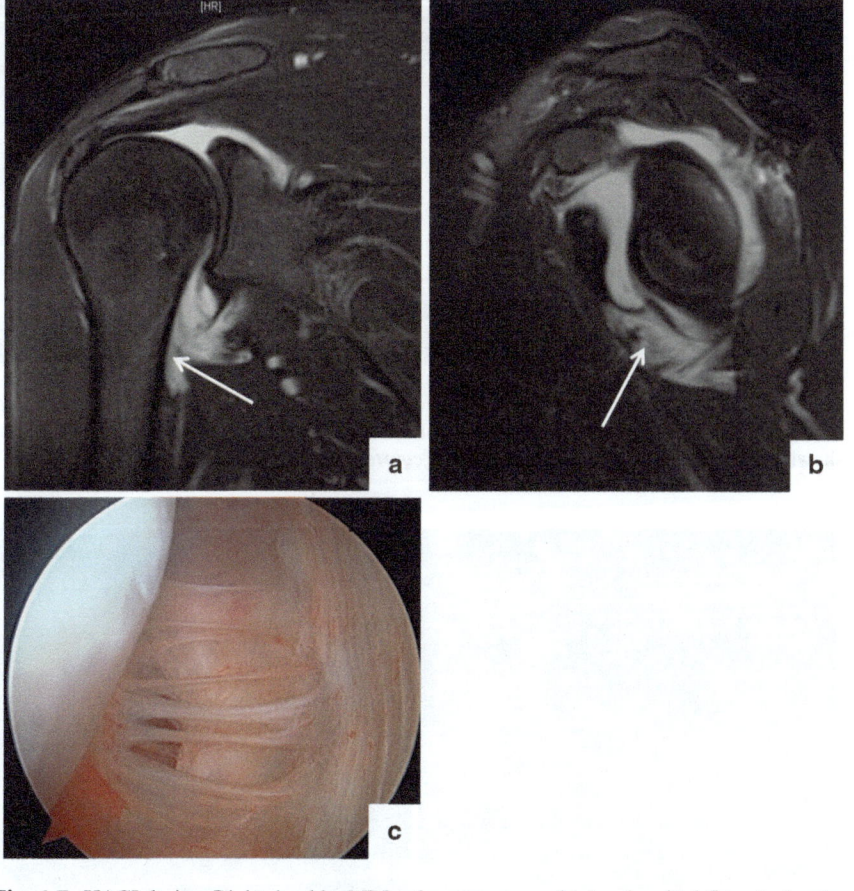

Fig. 1.7 HAGL lesion. Right shoulder MRI arthrogram coronal (**a**) and sagittal (**b**) cuts showing large glenohumeral ligament avulsion from the humerus (*arrows*). **c** Arthroscopy photo from same patient demonstrating large disruption of the glenohumeral ligament complex from the humerus (*Pictures courtesy* of Dr. Alison Toth)

The CT scan can also help with characterization of a Hill-Sachs lesion or with greater tuberosity fractures [34].

1.4   Indications and Contraindications for Surgical Stabilization

Though this is an area of long standing controversy, multiple studies have shown that young males are good candidates for surgical stabilization for anterior traumatic instability because they have high rates of recurrent dislocation. The decision to surgically intervene is on an individual patient basis. There is no infallible

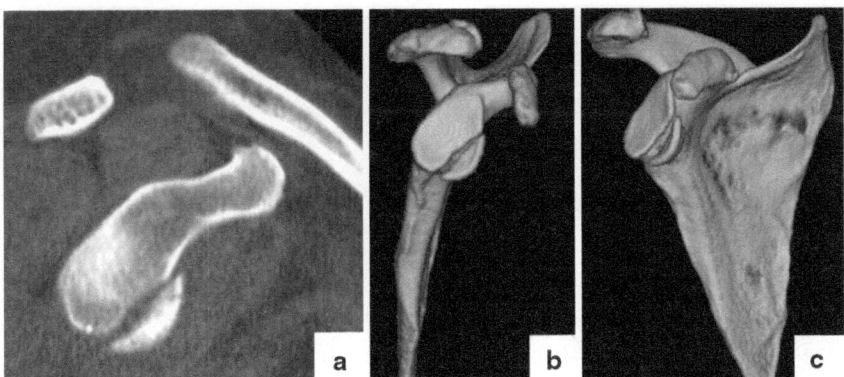

Fig. 1.8 CT scan right shoulder with large glenoid fragment. **a** 2D CT showing large anterior inferior glenoid fragment. **b/c** 3D CT scans help more clearly define size, shape, and location of glenoid fragment in preparation for repair. In this case, fragment is greater than 25 % of glenoid

Table 1.2 Factors for consideration in operative versus non-operative care of the first-time anterior dislocation

Objective Considerations	Subjective Considerations
Age	WOSI Components:
Sex	Physical symptoms of instability/pain
Contact vs. Non-contact Athlete	Limitations in work/recreation/sport
Mid-season athletic injury	Limitations to normal lifestyle activities
Overhead occupation (ex. Painter)	(ex. sleeping/fear of falling on shoulder)
	Emotional toll from instability
	(ex. Frustration from instability)

decision making plan for this injury, however, there are sufficient data to support early surgical stabilization following first-time traumatic anterior shoulder dislocation. The decision to operate should be based on many factors including age, activity level, work status (overhead versus non-overhead), potential for lost wages, contact sport participation, and ability of the patient to cope with the instability (Table 1.2).

While surgical stabilization for traumatic anterior instability remains elective, surgery is strongly recommended in several situations. We feel surgery should be considered non-elective and urgent if there is an irreducible dislocation (e.g. perched dislocation Fig. 1.9), fracture requiring surgical stabilization (e.g. a displaced greater tuberosity fracture), non-concentric glenohumeral reduction, or tissue interposition blocking adequate reduction. Similarly, surgery should be strongly recommended in the setting of a humeral head articular defect of >25 % or with an associated rotator cuff tear (>50 % cuff tear). If the dislocation occurs during the season for a high level athlete, the inability to participate in normal sports specific drills with intention to return to sport in the future would be another strong

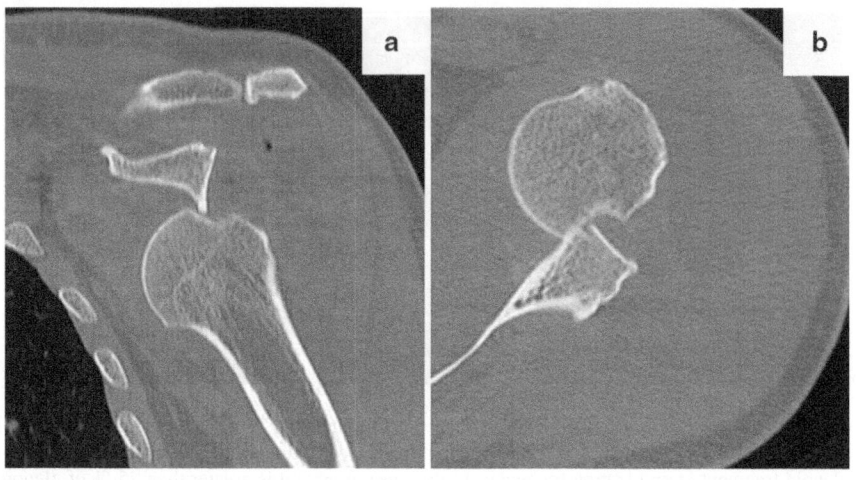

Fig. 1.9 Irreducible, perched, engaged Hill-Sachs lesion from left shoulder dislocation requiring surgical relocation. **a** Coronal CT. **b** Axial CT (*Picture courtesy* of Dr. Grant Garrigues)

indication for surgery. Relative indications for surgery include multiple dislocations within the same athletic season, contact sports activity, and age <20 years [19].

There are few contraindications to early surgical stabilization of a first-time shoulder dislocation, but surgery should be avoided if it is felt that the patient will be unable to comply with postoperative rehabilitation and restrictions. Similarly, a patient with significant medical co-morbidities limiting surgical intervention or post-operative rehabilitation should not undergo surgical stabilization due to associated risks and complications.

1.5   Author's Preferred Surgical Technique

1.5.1   Patient Positioning

While there is disagreement over the benefits of open versus arthroscopic stabilization [16], the author's preferred treatment method, if possible, is arthroscopic for a Bankart lesion (involving less than 25 % of the glenoid if bony). Even if an open stabilization is indicated, a diagnostic arthroscopic evaluation of the glenohumeral joint can be helpful to visualize shoulder anatomy, specifically areas that are more difficult to visualize and repair using an open technique, such as superior labral tears or detachments.

For most instability cases, we prefer the lateral decubitus position (Fig. 1.10) The sitting position is a viable option as well that allows for easier conversion to a deltopectoral approach if open surgery is indicated (Fig. 1.11). The lateral decubitus position allows for traction and abduction to be easily applied allowing for improved visualization of the joint space as well as access to the glenoid and labrum.

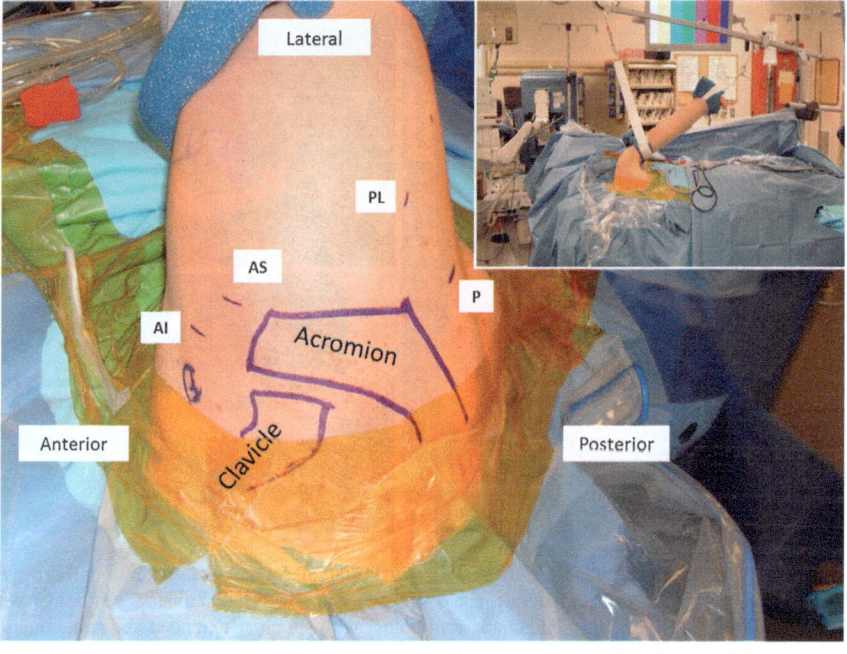

Fig. 1.10 Patient positioning and portal placement. Right shoulder in lateral decubitus position (*inset photo*) with *AI* (anterior inferior), *AS* (anterior superior), *PL* (posterolateral), and *P* (posterior) portals

After induction of general or regional anesthesia, a thorough examination under anesthesia (EUA) is performed. The patient is placed in the lateral decubitus position, supported by a beanbag. (Inset picture, Fig. 1.10) EUA includes assessing range of motion, as well as anterior, posterior, and inferior load-and-shift tests. The shoulder and upper extremity are then prepped and draped in sterile fashion. The upper extremity is placed in traction and approximately 40° of abduction. The placement for each portal is visualized in Fig. 1.10. A standard posterior portal is made, and a full diagnostic arthroscopy is performed. Anterior superior and anterior inferior portals are routinely utilized. The arthroscope should routinely be placed in the anterior superior portal (ASP) for further evaluation of the glenohumeral joint. The posterior labrum, glenoid cartilage, and glenohumeral ligaments are often better visualized through the ASP. Viewing from the ASP will also help avoid missing a HAGL or other associated ligamentous injury.

1.5.2 Soft Tissue Bankart Repair

Soft tissue Bankart repair requires careful soft tissue handling and good suture management. When the capsulolabral complex is located, it must be elevated and mobilized off the glenoid neck. After this tissue is free, the glenoid edge should be

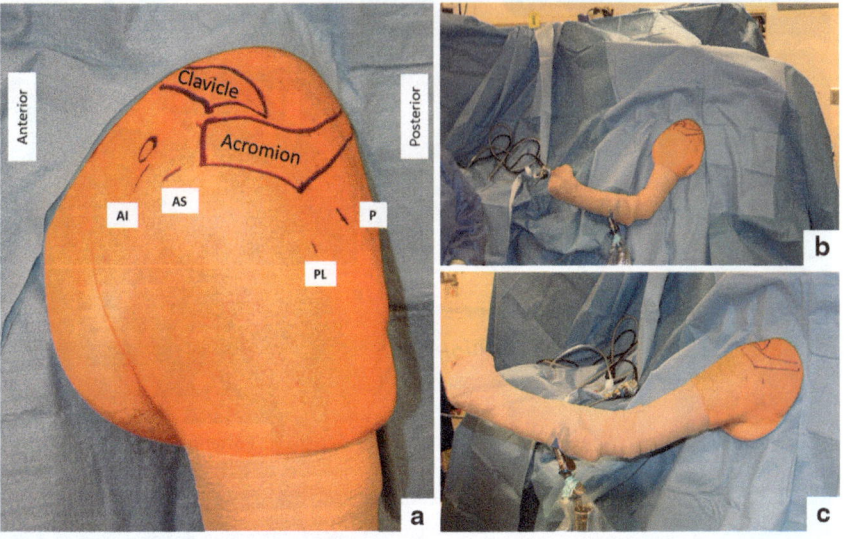

Fig. 1.11 Sitting position setup, left shoulder. **a** Portal placement: *AI* (anterior inferior), *AS* (anterior superior), *PL* (posterolateral), and *P* (posterior) portals. **b** Pneumatic arm holder with elbow at 90 degrees flexion. **c** Pneumatic arm holder with shoulder extended and some traction allowing similar access to labrum as lateral decubitus traction position

cleared of any scar tissue. The glenoid rim and scapular neck are then abraded with an arthroscopic rasp, shaver, or burr to create a bleeding healing surface. Avoid excessive bone removal and damage to the glenoid cartilage. Use a meniscal rasp to roughen the under surface of the freed labrum to promote healing.

Next, careful anchor placement is completed along the glenoid face. Anchors are placed 1-2 mm onto the articular cartilage surface. If the glenoid is pictured as a clock face, usually one anchor is utilized for each number on the clock face where the labrum is being repaired to the glenoid. Positioning the anchor too far medially will malreduce the labrum off the glenoid. Positioning too far onto the glenoid articular margin risks skiving under the cartilage and creation of a chondral flap. The anchor trochar is placed approximately 45° to the surface of the glenoid. It is important to appreciate that when placing anchors in various aspects of the glenoid, different angles of insertion and location with respect to the glenoid face are utilized (Fig. 1.12). For example, an anterior labral repair is more of a bumper than a posterior labral repair, and hence anchors needs to be placed further onto the glenoid rim.

While there are different ways to pass sutures from the anchor through the detached capsulolabral complex, we usually use a curved suture lasso or suture hook to pass sutures. Capsular redundancy can be addressed by passing the sutures separately through the capsule and the labrum. This effectively creates tucks in the capsular tissue that ultimately results in a tighter repair and decreased humeral head translation. Once the suture has been shuttled through the capsulolabral

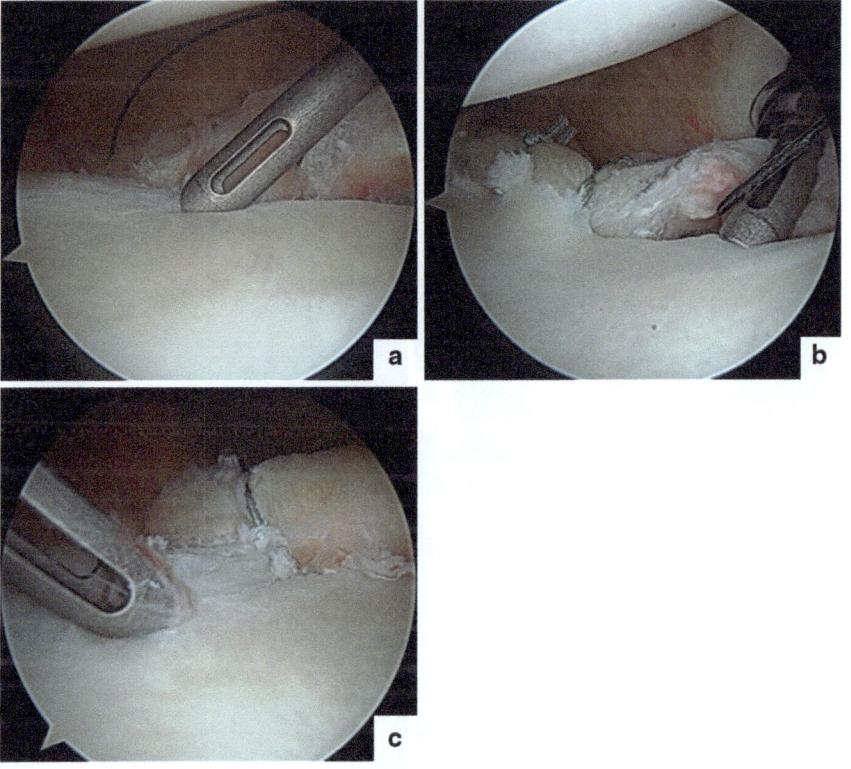

Fig. 1.12 Location for anchor placement for different parts of the glenoid/labrum for a left shoulder in the lateral decubitus position. **a** Posterior portal viewing placement of anterior inferior anchor (7 o'clock position) 1 mm onto the glenoid articular cartilage to help secure anterior-inferior "bumper". **b** Posterior portal viewing placement of anterior superior anchor (10:30 position) on the edge of the glenoid face. **c** Posterior portal viewing placement of posterior inferior anchor (near 6 o'clock position) just off articular cartilage face

tissue, a grasper is used to hold the repair tissue reduced in the planned fixation location with appropriate tension on the capsule. The sutures are tied arthroscopically using sliding locking knots. All knots are kept as far from the articular margin as possible to avoid irritation and cartilage scuffing. Finally, humeral head translation is assessed under direct visualization of the repaired tissue. While we use suture anchors and non-absorbable sutures, knotless anchors, absorbable sutures, or both also work well [35, 36].

1.5.3 Bony Bankart Repair

For bony Bankart lesions, the bony fragment is isolated and mobilized with arthroscopic elevators. Typically, the fragment is depressed medially from the

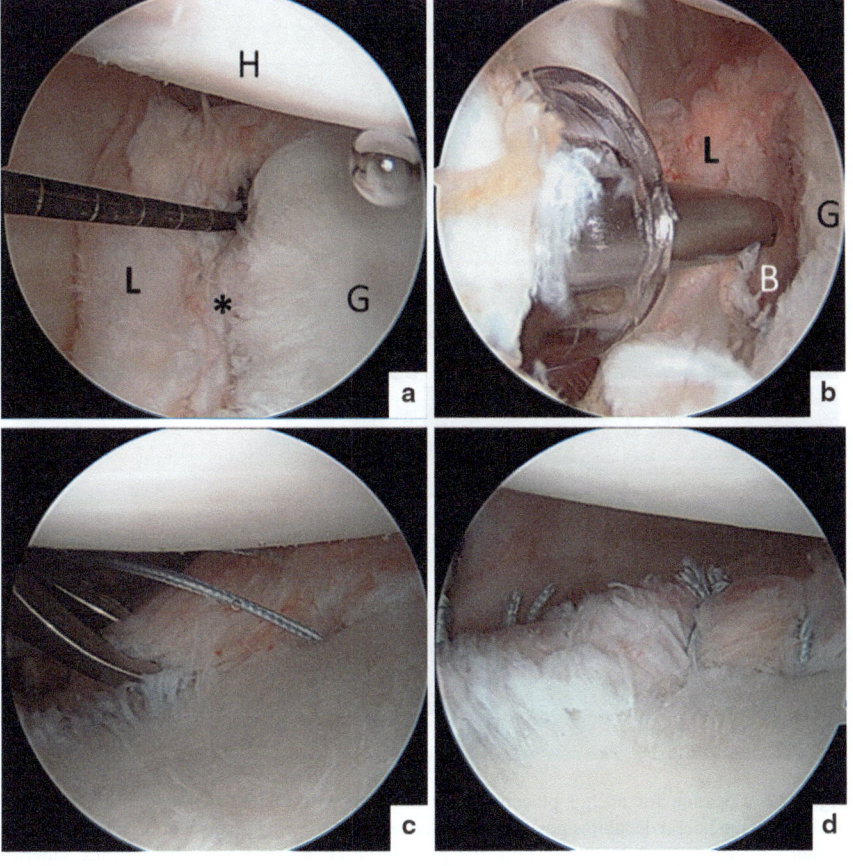

Fig. 1.13 Bony Bankart repair in right shoulder in lateral decubitus position. **a** Bony Bankart fragment (*) attached to labrum (*L*), scarred medially off glenoid (*G*) face. **b** Elevated bony bankart (*B*) with labrum (*L*). Abrasion of glenoid (*G*) edge promotes healing. **c** Suture from suture anchor around capsulolabral complex. Grasper used to pull tissue up to final attachment position. **d** Completed Bankart repair. Sutures off glenoid face

normal glenoid, separated by a scar tissue layer. Care should be taken not to damage the bony fragment, as it can be quite thin. It is often useful to keep this fragment for bone-on-bone healing with the repair; however, if the fragment is very small, it can be excised. Once the fragment is free, the repair technique mirrors that of the soft tissue Bankart. The surgeon should make effort to bring the bone up to its original location while still creating a good bumper with the capsulolabral complex. Finally, shoulder stability is tested under direct visualization of the repaired tissue. A case demonstrating bony Bankart repair is shown in Fig. 1.13.

1.5.4 HAGL Lesion

The HAGL lesion can be treated arthroscopically or open. We find that an arthroscopically assisted open procedure yields the most optimal results. The sitting position is used with a pneumatic arm holder (Fig. 1.11). The arthroscopic portion of the procedure allows for adequate visualization of the glenohumeral joint and other possible pathology. A thorough inspection of the entirety of the axillary pouch and humeral attachments of the glenohumeral ligaments can be done. Identification of the precise location for repair anchors and all necessary debridement is done arthroscopically.

The deltopectoral approach is utilized. The most critical aspect of this open procedure is preservation of the superior portion of the subscapularis muscle attachment. Expose the HAGL lesion by making an L-shaped incision starting on the inferior portion of the subscapularis tendon about 1.5 cm medial to the lesser tuberosity [37]. The vertical limb of the L-shaped incision ends inferiorly just proximal to the anterior circumflex vessels. At this point, the horizontal section of the incision is made. Care must be taken to palpate for the axillary nerve to avoid injury. The tendon is tagged with suture and retracted superiorly to expose the HAGL lesion.

The avulsed glenohumeral ligaments are then located and prepared for reattachment via suture anchors into the humeral neck. The humeral side of the repair is debrided down to bleeding bone to improve healing. Typically, two to three suture anchors are needed to apply appropriate tension to the repair. A mattress suture pattern is employed. The subscapularis is then repaired, and soft tissue closure completed.

1.5.5 Closure of Rotator Interval Capsular Openings

Rarely in first-time traumatic dislocator does repair of the Bankart lesion or other offending pathology (e.g. HAGL lesion) results in continued instability. Hence, it is necessary to consider closure of the rotator interval capsular openings (RICO), often referred to as "rotator interval closure". The rotator interval is the area located between the supraspinatus tendon and the subscapularis tendon. We use the term "closure of the RICO's" to avoid confusion with closure of the rotator interval, which implies plication of the subscapularis to the supraspinatus [38]. DePalma et al. classified the variable anatomy of the anterior capsular tissue into six groups based on the presence/absence and morphology of the foramen of Weitbracht (capsular opening superolateral to the middle glenohumeral ligament) and the foramen of Rouviere (capsular opening inferomedial to the middle glenohumeral ligament) [39]. DePalma called these foramen "synovial recesses". We agree with the findings of Provencher et al. which suggest that anterior translation and external rotation are limited by closure of the foramen of Weitbracht (imbrication of the middle glenohumeral ligament to the superior glenohumeral ligament), and that any posterior translation is not addressed with closure of the RICOs [40]. In cases of anterior instability, RICO closure may be added to reduce anterior humeral head translation following labral repair if there is concern about excess anterior laxity/anterior capsular redundancy, or in capsulorrhaphy procedures in shoulder with an intact labrum.

RICO closure can be done several different ways. With the arthroscope in the posterior portal, the anterior shoulder can be visualized. The anterior superior cannula is carefully pulled just outside the capsule. A penetrator with a number 2 non-absorbable suture is passed through the middle glenohumeral ligament near the superior border of the subscapularis tendon. The suture is pulled into the joint, and the penetrator is then again passed into the joint. This time, it pierces the superior glenohumeral ligament. An arthroscopic knot is the tied. Alternatively, a suture hook can be used via the anterior superior portal. This requires suture shuttling, but is also very effective.

1.6   Postoperative Rehabilitation Protocol

Following arthroscopic stabilization, the patient is placed into a shoulder immobilizer. We have a postoperative protocol with three distinct phases working towards full return to activity. Stage I is from 0 to 6 weeks postoperatively. For the first four weeks, the patient remains in the shoulder immobilizer. During this time, scapular stabilization, supported pendulum, and internal and external rotation exercises with the arm at the side are done under direct supervision of a physical therapy team. We routinely use water therapy between two and four weeks postoperatively (when wounds are healed) to work on early range of motion. Between four and six weeks postoperatively, the patient can discontinue sling wear as comfort allows.

Stage II is from 6 to 12 weeks after surgery. The goals of this phase are to gently increase glenohumeral range of motion, minimize shoulder pain, and progress from active- assist motion to active motion. Stage III (3 to 6 months postoperative) focuses on maximizing the strength of shoulder stabilizers, functional training for safe return to sport or work activity, and full range of motion. Most patients return to full activity at approximately six months.

1.7   Complications

There are several potential complications of traumatic anterior shoulder dislocations. In addition, there are several potential complications associated with surgical stabilization. Following dislocation, approximately 20–50 % of patients will have some type of neurologic complication [29]. For example, Visser et al. showed that 42 % of 77 patients with anterior dislocations had electromyographic evidence of axillary nerve damage [29]. For the most part, this is a stretch-induced neuropraxia. Other commonly injured nerves include the suprascapular, musculocutaneous, and radial nerves.

Two avoidable errors in managing shoulder dislocations remain failure to get adequate imaging to identify the dislocation (often from poor imaging due to patient discomfort) and failure to radiographically confirm reduction. Identifying fractures associated with dislocation is also critical. Missing a greater tuberosity fracture on X-ray may cause significant disability if the bone heals with the rotator cuff musculature in a shortened position.

In general, surgical complication rates for open and arthroscopic shoulder instability surgery are low. Kang et al. grouped the surgical complications into perioperative, intraoperative, and postoperative complications [41]. Perioperative complications include misdiagnosis, inadequate imaging, inadequate history and physical, and failure to identify concomitant injuries. It is critical that the surgeon know the nature of the dislocation and the associated physical exam limitations that may indicate other pathologic changes such as rotator cuff or superior labral tears [21, 42, 43].

Intraoperative complications include nerve injury, failure to appropriately tension the repair, misdiagnosis of the injury causing the instability, and hardware failure. The most commonly injured nerves in open and arthroscopic instability repair remain the axillary and musculocutaneous nerves, mostly from improper retraction and excessive traction [44–46]. Tensioning the repair can be very difficult, especially if there is significant scaring of the labrum to the medial glenoid and capsular contraction. If the humeral head translation cannot be adequately controlled, even with significant tension on the repair, look for other possible injuries such as glenohumeral ligament disruption. Similarly, if the patient continues to have anterior inferior translation with the arm in adduction, capsular plication and possible RICO closure should be considered. Hardware failure is uncommon. It is important that anchors are firmly secured within the bone and are not placed too flat relative to the cartilage surface. This can lead to chondral injury and failure.

Finally, postoperative complications include stiffness, pain, infection, and recurrence. Stiffness can occur as a function of over-tightening of the anterior capsule or as an adhesive capsulitis. Both of these are rare, and therapy can help prevent these entities. Most importantly, we recommend that therapy not be done beyond the point of discomfort. Aggressive physical therapy inducing significant pain is likely to cause increased stiffness and irritation to the joint, which is counterproductive. Infection after instability surgery is very uncommon. A 20-year series from the Mayo Clinic identified only six infections from instability surgeries. [47] Despite different treatment modes for the instability used in the Mayo Clinic study, the recommendations remained the same including appreciation of both early (<6 weeks) or late (>8 months) infections, as well as culturing for Proprionobacterium acnes when working up all infections. Recurrence rates vary within the literature following stabilization. One recent systematic review [13] and one evidenced-based medicine review [48] suggest recurrence rates after surgery between 3 and 20 %. The increased likelihood of injury is associated with young age and higher activity levels.

1.8 Conclusion

Traumatic anterior shoulder instability is a common and complex problem facing the orthopaedic surgeon. This injury can result in significant disability and time lost from work or sport. Early operative stabilization in young patients is associated with improved clinical outcomes over non-operative treatment. Decision Analysis Modeling continues to improve the surgeon's ability to predict outcomes while allowing the patient to participate in the decision to treat this injury operatively or non-operatively. With good data to support these models, the discussion between patient and surgeon can now be done with more information to help project successful outcomes based on patient specific factors, leading to more optimal outcomes and patient satisfaction.

References

1. Boileau P, Walch G (1997) The three-dimensional geometry of the proximal humerus. Implications for surgical technique and prosthetic design. J Bone Joint Surg Br 79(5):857–865
2. Churchill RS, Brems JJ, Kotschi H (2001) Glenoid size, inclination, and version: an anatomic study. J Shoulder Elbow Surg 10(4):327–332 PubMed PMID: 11517362
3. Turkel SJ, Panio MW, Marshall JL, Girgis FG (1981) Stabilizing mechanisms preventing anterior dislocation of the glenohumeral joint. J Bone Joint Surg Am 63(8):1208–1217
4. Bankart AS (1923) Recurrent or habitual dislocation of the shoulder-joint. Br Med J 2(3285):1132–1133
5. Taylor DC, Arciero RA (1997) Pathologic changes associated with shoulder dislocations. Arthroscopic and physical examination findings in first-time, traumatic anterior dislocations. Am J Sports Med 25(3):306–311 PubMed PMID: 9167808
6. Burkhart SS, De Beer JF (2000) Traumatic glenohumeral bone defects and their relationship to failure of arthroscopic Bankart repairs: significance of the inverted-pear glenoid and the humeral engaging Hill-Sachs lesion. Arthroscopy 16(7):677–694
7. Hill HA, Sachs MD (1940) The grooved defect of the humeral head: a frequently unrecongized complication of dislocations of the shoulder joint. Radiology 35:690–700
8. George MS, Khazzam M, Kuhn JE (2011) Humeral avulsion of glenohumeral ligaments. J Am Acad Orthop Surg. Mar;19(3):127–133 PubMed PMID: 21368093
9. Wolf EM, Cheng JC, Dickson K (1995) Humeral avulsion of glenohumeral ligaments as a cause of anterior shoulder instability. Arthroscopy 11(5):600–607
10. Wolf EM, Siparsky PN (2010) Glenoid avulsion of the glenohumeral ligaments as a cause of recurrent anterior shoulder instability. Arthroscopy 26(9):1263–1267 PubMed PMID: 20810083
11. Bokor DJ, Conboy VB, Olson C (1999) Anterior instability of the glenohumeral joint with humeral avulsion of the glenohumeral ligament. A review of 41 cases. J Bone Joint Surg Br 81(1):93–96
12. Bottoni CR, Wilckens JH, DeBerardino TM, D'Alleyrand JC, Rooney RC, Harpstrite JK et al (2002) A prospective, randomized evaluation of arthroscopic stabilization versus nonoperative treatment in patients with acute, traumatic, first-time shoulder dislocations. Am J Sports Med 30(4):576–580 PubMed PMID: 12130413
13. Brophy RH, Marx RG (2009) The treatment of traumatic anterior instability of the shoulder: nonoperative and surgical treatment. Arthroscopy 25(3):298–304

14. Handoll HH, Almaiyah MA, Rangan A (2004) Surgical versus non-surgical treatment for acute anterior shoulder dislocation. Cochrane Database Syst Rev 2004(1):CD004325 PubMed PMID: 14974064
15. Hovelius L, Augustini BG, Fredin H, Johansson O, Norlin R, Thorling J (1996) Primary anterior dislocation of the shoulder in young patients. A ten-year prospective study. J Bone Joint Surg Am 78(11):1677–1684
16. Jakobsen BW, Johannsen HV, Suder P, Sojbjerg JO (2007) Primary repair versus conservative treatment of first-time traumatic anterior dislocation of the shoulder: a randomized study with 10-year follow-up. Arthroscopy 23(2):118–123
17. Kirkley A, Werstine R, Ratjek A, Griffin S (2005) Prospective randomized clinical trial comparing the effectiveness of immediate arthroscopic stabilization versus immobilization and rehabilitation in first traumatic anterior dislocations of the shoulder: long-term evaluation. Arthroscopy 21(1):55–63
18. Mather RC 3rd, Orlando LA, Henderson RA, Lawrence JT, Taylor DC (2011) A predictive model of shoulder instability after a first-time anterior shoulder dislocation. J Shoulder Elbow Surg 20(2):259–266 PubMed PMID: 21276928
19. Owens BD, Agel J, Mountcastle SB, Cameron KL, Nelson BJ (2009) Incidence of glenohumeral instability in collegiate athletics. Am J Sports Med 37(9):1750–1754
20. Owens BD, Dawson L, Burks R, Cameron KL (2009) Incidence of shoulder dislocation in the United States military: demographic considerations from a high-risk population. J Bone Joint Surg Am 91(4):791–796
21. Owens BD, Duffey ML, Nelson BJ, DeBerardino TM, Taylor DC, Mountcastle SB (2007) The incidence and characteristics of shoulder instability at the United States Military Academy. Am J Sports Med 35(7):1168–1173
22. Porcellini G, Paladini P, Campi F, Paganelli M (2007) Long-term outcome of acute versus chronic bony Bankart lesions managed arthroscopically. Am J Sports Med 35(12):2067–2072
23. Robinson CM, Howes J, Murdoch H, Will E, Graham C (2006) Functional outcome and risk of recurrent instability after primary traumatic anterior shoulder dislocation in young patients. J Bone Joint Surg Am 88(11):2326–2336
24. Robinson CM, Jenkins PJ, White TO, Ker A, Will E (2008) Primary arthroscopic stabilization for a first-time anterior dislocation of the shoulder. A randomized, double-blind trial. J Bone Joint Surg Am 90(4):708–721
25. Sachs RA, Lin D, Stone ML, Paxton E, Kuney M (2007) Can the need for future surgery for acute traumatic anterior shoulder dislocation be predicted? J Bone Joint Surg Am 89(8):1665–1674 PubMed PMID: 17671003
26. te Slaa RL, Wijffels MP, Brand R, Marti RK (2004) The prognosis following acute primary glenohumeral dislocation. J Bone Joint Surg Br 86(1):58–64
27. Wheeler JH, Ryan JB, Arciero RA, Molinari RN (1989) Arthroscopic versus nonoperative treatment of acute shoulder dislocations in young athletes. Arthroscopy 5(3):213–217
28. Plancher KD, Lipnick SL (2009) Analysis of evidence-based medicine for shoulder instability. Arthroscopy 25(8):897–908
29. Visser CP, Coene LN, Brand R, Tavy DL (1999) The incidence of nerve injury in anterior dislocation of the shoulder and its influence on functional recovery. A prospective clinical and EMG study. J Bone Joint Surg Br 81(4):679–685
30. Bahk M, Keyurapan E, Tasaki A, Sauers EL, McFarland EG (2007) Laxity testing of the shoulder: a review. Am J Sports Med 35(1):131–144
31. Farber AJ, Castillo R, Clough M, Bahk M, McFarland EG (2006) Clinical assessment of three common tests for traumatic anterior shoulder instability. J Bone Joint Surg Am 88(7):1467–1474
32. Greenspan A (2004) Orthopedic imaging: a practical approach. Lippincott Williams & Wilkins, Philadelphia, p 98

33. Provencher MT, Ghodadra N, LeClere L, Solomon DJ, Romeo AA (2009) Anatomic osteochondral glenoid reconstruction for recurrent glenohumeral instability with glenoid deficiency using a distal tibia allograft. Arthroscopy 25(4):446–452

34. Provencher MT, Ghodadra N, Romeo AA (2010) Arthroscopic management of anterior instability: pearls, pitfalls, and lessons learned. Orthop Clin N Am 41(3):325–337

35. Monteiro GC, Ejnisman B, Andreoli CV, de Castro Pochini A, Cohen M (2008) Absorbable versus nonabsorbable sutures for the arthroscopic treatment of anterior shoulder instability in athletes: a prospective randomized study. Arthroscopy 24(6):697–703 PubMed PMID: 18514114

36. Oh JH, Lee HK, Kim JY, Kim SH, Gong HS (2009) Clinical and radiologic outcomes of arthroscopic glenoid labrum repair with the BioKnotless suture anchor. Am J Sports Med 37(12):2340–2348

37. Arciero RA, Mazzocca AD (2005) Mini-open repair technique of HAGL (humeral avulsion of the glenohumeral ligament) lesion. Arthroscopy 21(9):1152

38. Wilson WR, Magnussen RA, Irribarra LA, Taylor DC (2012) Variability of the capsular anatomy in the rotator interval region of the shoulder. J Shoulder Elbow Surg PubMed PMID: 23177168

39. DePalma A, Callery G, Bennett GA (1949) Variational anatomy and degenerative lesions of the shoulder joint. Instr Course Lect 6:255–281

40. Provencher MT, Mologne TS, Hongo M, Zhao K, Tasto JP, An KN (2007) Arthroscopic versus open rotator interval closure: biomechanical evaluation of stability and motion. Arthroscopy 23(6):583–592

41. Kang RW, Frank RM, Nho SJ, Ghodadra NS, Verma NN, Romeo AA et al (2009) Complications associated with anterior shoulder instability repair. Arthroscopy 25(8):909–920

42. Owens BD, Nelson BJ, Duffey ML, Mountcastle SB, Taylor DC, Cameron KL et al (2010) Pathoanatomy of first-time, traumatic, anterior glenohumeral subluxation events. J Bone Joint Surg Am 92(7):1605–1611 PubMed PMID: 20595566

43. Tischer T, Vogt S, Kreuz PC, Imhoff AB (2011) Arthroscopic anatomy, variants, and pathologic findings in shoulder instability. Arthroscopy 27(10):1434–1443 PubMed PMID: 21871774

44. Boardman ND 3rd, Cofield RH (1999) Neurologic complications of shoulder surgery. Clin Orthop Relat Res 368:44–53

45. McFarland EG, Caicedo JC, Guitterez MI, Sherbondy PS, Kim TK (2001) The anatomic relationship of the brachial plexus and axillary artery to the glenoid. Implications for anterior shoulder surgery. Am J Sports Med 29(6):729–733 PubMed PMID: 11734485

46. Ho E, Cofield RH, Balm MR, Hattrup SJ, Rowland CM (1999) Neurologic complications of surgery for anterior shoulder instability. J Shoulder Elbow Surg 8(3):266–270 PubMed PMID: 10389084

47. Sperling JW, Cofield RH, Torchia ME, Hanssen AD (2003) Infection after shoulder instability surgery. Clin Orthop Relat Res 414:61–64

48. Kuhn JE (2006) Treating the initial anterior shoulder dislocation–an evidence-based medicine approach. Sports Med Arthrosc 14(4):192–198

Management of Shoulder Instability in the Collision Athlete

2

A Technique-Based Review, Focusing on the Indications, Evaluation, Techniques, Outcomes, and Evidence on this Topic in the Area of Shoulder Instability Surgery

Matthew A. Cavagnaro and Steven B. Cohen

2.1 Evaluation of the Collision Athlete with Shoulder Instability

2.1.1 History

Evaluation of any athlete with a shoulder injury begins with a thorough history. The clinician should identify the onset, mechanism of injury, type of symptoms, and previous injuries. The collision athlete will often note onset associated with an acute event [4]. An anterior-to-posterior directed force to the upper arm while the arm is in abduction and external rotation represents the most common mechanism in an initial and/or recurrent traumatic anterior instability event. Tackling in American football or rugby, or landing on the field with the arm in this position can re-create this mechanism [1]. Other athletes may not recall a specific injury that produced their symptoms. They will not describe a dislocation event, but rather episodes where the arm "goes dead," feels heavy or weak, or that they feel a sharp posterior shoulder pain after forced external rotation in the overhead position. These symptoms should raise suspicion for shoulder subluxation. In this case, the athlete is often unaware of the abnormal movement of the shoulder [4]. For the contact athlete who describes symptoms of instability, but has no history of injury or association of symptoms with collisions, an underlying diagnosis of multi-directional instability (MDI) should be considered. These patients will often have bilateral symptoms. Although the vast majority of collision athletes with shoulder instability result from trauma, patients with generalized laxity at risk for MDI also participate in these sports, and this is important to consider as treatment will often

M. A. Cavagnaro · S. B. Cohen (✉)
Director of Sports Medicine Research, Department of Orthopaedic Surgery, Thomas Jefferson University, Rothman Institute Sports Medicine, 925 Chestnut St. 5th Floor, Philadelphia, PA 19107-4216, USA
e-mail: steven.cohen@rothmaninstitute.com

S. F. Brockmeier et al. (eds.), *Surgery of Shoulder Instability*,
DOI: 10.1007/978-3-642-38100-3_2, © ISAKOS 2013

23

vary [5]. Pain associated with anterior instability is usually sharp and occurs in the region of the posterior capsule when the shoulder is abducted and externally rotated [4]. Asking the patient about previous injuries and surgical procedures is important. For patients with a formal dislocation, the number of dislocation events, treatments (both non-surgical and surgical), and the mechanisms causing the dislocations are all very important when taking a history. This information can help in several ways. Knowing whether the patient is a first time dislocator versus recurrent dislocator will often affect further workup and management. If they've had prior treatments that have now failed, future management options will be affected. Often recurrent dislocators will describe instability episodes that tend to occur with less energy at less extremes of motion, which could result from bone loss, and will help to guide further workup and management.

2.1.2 Physical Examination

A number of shoulder pathologies are common in athletes, and for that reason, a thorough shoulder examination including inspection, palpation, and range of motion testing in both the injured and asymptomatic shoulders should be done in all athletes presenting with shoulder pain. Specific to shoulder instability patients, a patient with an acute glenohumeral dislocation will often have a palpable prominence of the humeral head anterior and inferior to the shoulder, as well as a lack of shoulder contour over the deltoid. The arm is generally held in a position of adduction and internal rotation, and abduction of the arm is limited to <90° [2]. In patients who present after relocation, one should look for previous surgical scars, and compare both sides to look for muscle atrophy, or scapular winging that could signify nerve injury. Nerve injuries associated with shoulder dislocation include axillary nerve, suprascapular nerve traction, and the long thoracic nerve, with axillary nerve injury reported to be as high as 42 % based on electromyography (EMG) findings [1, 6]. Range of motion (ROM) examination can help ensure glenohumeral reduction. A complete neurovascular exam including strength testing of the deltoid and external rotators can assess axillary and suprascapular nerve function. In patients that have had prior open surgery, it's important to test subscapularis function as failure of prior repair can occur [7].

The mainstay of the physical exam for patients with suspected shoulder instability involves special tests aimed at characterizing the shoulder instability pattern. These tests include sulcus sign, apprehension, relocation, surprise, jerk, and load-and-shift tests. Comparing the symptomatic and normal shoulders can help quantify the direction and magnitude of laxity. Upon completion of these tests, the clinician should have identified those with MDI versus unidirectional instability. In those with unidirectional instability, the direction and magnitude of instability should be identified [7].

The sulcus sign provides an objective measure of inferior glenohumeral laxity and is often present in patients with generalized laxity at risk for MDI. The test is performed with the patient in the seated or supine position with the arm in neutral position. Longitudinal inferior traction is applied to the humerus, and the distance from the humerus to the acromion is evaluated. A 1+ sulcus sign represents 1 cm of inferior translation, and signs of 2+ and 3+ represent 2 and 3 cm of translation, respectively [2]. A 2+ or greater score is considered a high degree of glenohumeral laxity, but is only considered abnormal in the symptomatic patient [8]. The same test is performed again with the arm in 30° of external rotation. A sign that persists in external rotation suggests incompetence of the superior glenohumeral ligament and rotator interval. Elimination of the sulcus sign in this position suggests a competent rotator interval [2].

The apprehension, relocation, and surprise tests assess for anterior instability. The apprehension test is performed with the patient seated or supine. The shoulder is abducted 90° and externally rotated with gentle anterior force. Guarding or apprehension during this maneuver indicates a positive test. Pain without apprehension is not considered a positive test, but may indicate more subtle anterior instability [9, 10]. Often, patients with soft-tissue instability will experience apprehension at 90° abduction, but those patients with bony defects may experience apprehension in lower, or midrange (i.e., 20° to 60°), abduction angles [11]. The relocation test, described by Jobe et al. [12] is performed with the patient supine. With the arm in the apprehension test position, a posteriorly directed force on the humeral head that causes disappearance or improvement of symptoms is considered a positive result. Releasing this posteriorly directed force with immediate return of apprehension is considered a positive surprise test. The surprise test has been shown to be the most accurate individual test for anterior instability with a positive predictive value of 98 % and a negative predictive value of 78 % [2, 13].

Tests specific for assessing posterior instability include the posterior stress test, jerk test, and Kim test. The posterior stress test is performed with the individual in the supine position, with the arm flexed to 90° and internally rotated. The clinician axially loads the humerus against the posterior glenoid by pushing the arm posteriorly with one hand while the other hand supports the scapula posteriorly. This test is positive when a subluxation of the humeral head over the glenoid rim is palpated or observed [14]. The jerk test is performed with the patient seated and the examiner stands next to the affected shoulder, grasps the elbow with one hand and the distal clavicle and scapular spine in the other. After placing the arm in a flexed and internally rotated position, a posteriorly directed to the flexed elbow is applied while the shoulder girdle is pushed anteriorly. The test is positive when a sudden jerk associated with pain occurs as the subluxated humeral head relocates into the glenoid fossa [15]. The Kim test is performed with the patient seated and the arm in 90° abduction. The clinician grasps the elbow with one hand, with the other hand grasping the lateral aspect of the patient's proximal arm. While elevating the patient's arm to 45°, the clinician applies a downward and posterior force to the upper arm. A sudden onset of pain with this maneuver signifies a positive test [16, 17]. The combination of a positive jerk and Kim test has been shown to have 97 % sensitivity for posterior glenohumeral instability [17].

The load-and-shift test helps assess glenoid concavity and can be used to test for either anterior or posterior shoulder instability. Direction and degree of translation at different levels of glenohumeral abduction can be assessed with this test. With the patient seated or supine, and the arm in approximately 20° of forward flexion, the humeral head is loaded axially from the elbow while anterior and posterior stresses are applied to the proximal arm. This is often done at 0°, 45°, and 90° of abduction, and the direction and amount of translation is graded. Grade 1 represents increased translation compared to the normal side. Grade 2 indicates humeral head to, but not over, the glenoid rim while grade 3 is translation over the glenoid rim. Increased translation at higher degrees of abduction implies compromise of the inferior glenohumeral ligament (IGHL) [2]. The load-and-shift test has been shown to be up to 98 % specific, but has poor sensitivity for detecting glenohumeral instability [18].

2.1.3 Imaging

Radiographic evaluation of a patient with suspected glenohumeral instability should begin with quality plain radiographs. True anteroposterior (AP) (in the scapular plane), scapular Y, and axillary views can confirm reduction, reveal abnormal glenoid version, dysplasia, hypoplasia, or bone loss that may contribute to instability. A bony shadow or displaced bony Bankart fragment may be visualized on a true AP radiograph, however to better evaluate for an anterior glenoid defect, an apical oblique (West Point) view is more sensitive [19, 20]. The Stryker notch view and AP view in internal rotation can help evaluate potential Hill-Sachs lesions on the humerus [7, 21] Overall, plain radiographs have been found to be moderately accurate in demonstrating bone loss [22].

The current gold standard for pre-operative characterization and quantification of glenoid or humeral bone loss is computed tomography (CT). They can very accurately detect fracture fragments, and quantify bone loss. Glenoid osseous deficiency is quantified as a percentage of the normal inferior glenoid. A circle is drawn to fit the inferior two-thirds of the glenoid image, which is a consistent anatomic configuration [23]. Using digital measurements, the amount of bone missing from the total surface area of the inferior circle is calculated [7]. Concerning humeral bone loss, CT has been shown to provide enough detail to characterize the depth and orientation of Hill-Sachs lesions, which can help to determine if the lesion is likely to be an engaging defect [24]. Obtaining a CT scan should strongly be considered in any patient whose history, physical exam, or plain radiographs suggest bone loss.

Magnetic resonance imaging (MRI) has also shown high sensitivity and specificity for the detection of glenoid and humeral head bone defects, but the detail provided by CT is unmatched [10]. MRI does, however, provide excellent detail of soft tissue and is frequently used to evaluate patients with shoulder instability. Magnetic resonance arthrography (MRA) may be more useful than MRI because the capsule becomes distended improving definition of the glenoid labrum, rotator interval, and glenohumeral ligaments. In collision athletes, MRA can help identify Bankart lesions, ligamentous deficiencies/humeral avulsion of glenohumeral ligament (HAGL), patulous capsules, and other soft tissue pathologies [8].

2.2 Management of Shoulder Instability in the Collision Athlete

Decision-making in the management of collision athletes with shoulder instability must take several things into consideration. The overall goal of treatment is to return the athlete to competition safely and efficiently, however, there is often pressure to minimize time away from competition, to prevent further injury, and restore function. Criteria for in-season return to play following an initial acute shoulder instability event, as described by Owens et al. [2], include symmetric pain-free ROM and strength, ability to perform sport-specific skills, and the absence of subjective or objective instability. In deciding how best to manage shoulder instability in a collision athlete, one must consider timing within the competitive season, the likelihood of non-operative treatment allowing an early return, and the risks that may be involved with early return. Whether the patient has suffered an isolated instability event vs recurrence, if they have failed prior treatments, and the severity of instability at time of evaluation help to guide management decisions.

2.2.1 Nonoperative Treatment

Nonoperative treatment for shoulder instability in athletes includes immobilization, physical therapy, and bracing. While nonsurgical treatment is widely used, and has historically been the standard of treatment for acute first-time dislocation in athletes, this has recently been disputed. Kirkley et al. [25] showed a higher recurrence rate of instability with conservative treatment and improved quality of life with surgical treatment in the young athletic population. Nevertheless, nonoperative treatment remains a viable option and relative indications include first-time dislocation, osseous defects of the glenoid <25 %, osseous defects of the humeral head <25 % (Fig. 2.1), and absence of fracture or soft-tissue injury requiring surgery. Player specific indications include a desire to return to sport in-season, a non-overhead athlete, and the athlete can perform sport-specific drills without instability [2]. In athletes with these goals, nonoperative treatment may be a temporary measure with surgical management planned after the season, but the increased risk of recurrent instability must be communicated. Buss et al. [26] found that 27 of 30 patients (24 involved in collision sports) were able to return to their sport at subjectively the same level of play after nonoperative treatment of shoulder instability. Of those that returned, 26 were able to finish the season, however, 10 (37 %) experienced an episode of recurrent instability during the season. The average time missed from

Fig. 2.1 Hill-Sachs humeral
head defect

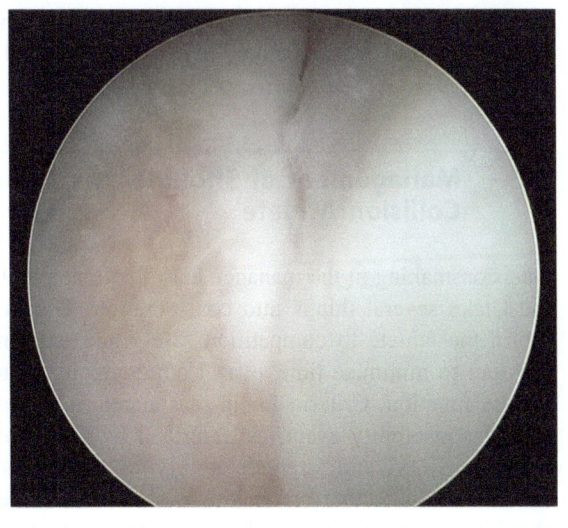

sport after the instability event in this study was 10.2 days, and 12 of these patients required surgical stabilization after the season.

Despite the evidence that nonoperative treatment can be effective in returning an athlete to competition in-season, several studies have shown that the young male athlete is most at risk for shoulder instability and recurrence with non-surgical treatment. One study reported a re-dislocation rate of 100 % in patients younger than 10 years, 94 % in 10–20 year-olds, and 79 % in 20–30 year-olds [31]. Robinson et al. [27] reported a recurrence rate of 87 % in patients aged 15–20 years treated non-surgically following anterior shoulder dislocation. Another study found the rate of recurrence to decrease with age at time of instability event. In this study, patients older than 30 years had a recurrence rate of 27 %, while those younger than 23 years had a 72 % rate of recurrence [32]. This information is important to consider when counseling a young athlete regarding risk of recurrence when returning them to sport in-season after non-surgical treatment.

The length of immobilization and position of immobilization following instability events in athletes has been an area of controversy. Traditionally, immobilization had been in a sling with the arm adducted and internally rotated. Recurrence rates following this type of immobilization in young athletes in collision sports have been reported to be as high as 90 % [28]. Itoi et al. [29], using MRI, found that immobilization in internal rotation displaces the labrum, while those immobilized in external rotation (mean 35°) had less separation and displacement of the labrum. In a follow-up study, they randomized 198 patients after an initial dislocation to either internal or external rotation immobilization and found the recurrent instability rate in the external rotation group to be significantly lower (26 %) than the internal rotation grough (42 %) [30]. In a more recent randomized controlled trial, however, these results could not be reproduced as immobilization in external rotation following initial dislocation did not reduce the recurrence rate [31].

Most studies have found duration of immobilization after an instability event does not have a significant affect on rate of recurrence. Hovelius et al. prospectively studied 257 patients treated with either shoulder immobilization in a sling for 3–4 weeks or freedom to use the shoulder as tolerated immediately after evaluation. The authors found no difference in redislocation rates between the two groups at 2-year follow-up [2, 32]. Several authors advocate early mobilization, and have found the rate of recurrent instability with non-surgical treatment to be related to age and not duration of immobilization [26].

Recommendations for rehabilitation prior to return-to-play after an episode of shoulder instability are fairly consistent. Whether or not a period of immobilization is utilized following an instability event, cryotherapy with early initiation of ROM exercises is recommended. As pain and ROM improve, the patient should progress to strengthening exercises focusing on the dynamic shoulder stabilizers. Resistance is graduated until the athlete displays symmetric shoulder and scapular strength. Lastly, sport-specific exercises are initiated and progressed until the athlete has no symptoms of instability or apprehension [26, 33].

Bracing for return-to-sport for shoulder instability has not been shown to decrease recurrence rate, although can be associated with subjective improvement in stability [2]. Bracing can range from motion-limiting braces that limit abduction, extension, and external rotation to neoprene sleeves. Collision athletes tend to tolerate the motion-limiting braces better than overhead athletes, and these may help provide an increased sense of stability and assist with return to play.

2.2.2   Risks Associated with Nonoperative Treatment

Nonoperative management for shoulder instability in collision athletes is associated with a high recurrence rate, as outlined above, and is well documented in the literature. What is not clearly defined is whether recurrent instability events are associated with worse overall functional outcomes. The concern is that recurrent instability events risks further damage to the labrum, articular cartilage, capsule, glenohumeral ligaments, glenoid, and humeral head [2].

The Bankart lesion, or detachment of the anteroinferior glenoid labrum and inferior glenohumeral ligament (IGHL) is the considered the predominant pathoanatomic lesion in traumatic anterior shoulder instability [34, 35]. Studies have found a Bankart lesion to be present in 79–100 % of patients after initial anterior dislocation, and in 93–97 % of those with recurrent dislocations [36–38]. These lesions are often associated with recurrent instability, and this data suggests there is a progressive pattern of injury to the soft-tissue restraints of the glenohumeral joint in patients with recurrent instability [1, 2, 39].

There also appears to be an association of recurrent instability and increased bone loss on both the humeral and glenoid sides. A Hill-Sachs lesion was present in 71–100 % of initial dislocations, however nearly all patients with recurrent instability have Hill-Sachs lesions [36, 40, 41]. Recurrence has also been associated with larger sized Hill-Sachs lesions, and engaging Hill-Sachs lesions [41]. Glenoid bone loss of <25 % has been identified in zero to 22 % of patients after initial dislocation, while 30–73 % of patients with recurrent instability patients exhibit this bone loss [1, 38, 40, 41]. Glenoid bone loss >25 % and the inverted-pear shaped glenoid has been found in 15–52 % of those with recurrent instability [24, 38, 41]. Given this data, it appears that recurrence of instability is not without risk of further damage to the natural anatomy of the shoulder. Without long-term prospective studies, however, we do not know what this may mean for functional outcomes.

2.2.3 Surgical Treatment

2.2.3.1 Indications
Management of a mid-season shoulder instability injury is complicated by return-to-play goals. Owens et al. [2] have outlined absolute and relative indications for early surgery in shoulder instability athletes. Absolute indications include: associated injuries, >50 % rotator cuff tear, glenoid osseous defect >25 %, humeral head articular surface osseous defect >25 %, proximal humerus fracture requiring surgery, irreducible dislocation, interposed tissue or nonconcentric reduction, failed trial of rehabilitation, inability to tolerate shoulder restrictions, and inability to perform sport-specific drills without instability. They identified relative indications include: >2 shoulder dislocations during the season, overhead throwing athletes, contact sport athletes, injury near the end of the season, and age <20 years. Collision athletes that lack an absolute indication for surgery are generally allowed a course of nonoperative treatment with early return to play. If surgery is indicated, this can be done after the season to limit time away from competition. If nonoperative treatment fails, the athlete should be taken out of competition and scheduled for surgical stabilization.

2.2.4 Open Versus Arthroscopic Stabilization

Until the late 1990s, arthroscopic treatment for shoulder instability in contact athletes was discredited when compared to open surgery. Several studies showed collision athletes to be at high risk for failure after arthroscopic stabilization procedures [42, 43, 44]. These publications included a wide variety of results with higher recurrence rates, different techniques, and different patient populations. They also did not take into account differing pathologic lesions [41]. Open stabilization was considered the gold standard for restoring shoulder stability in collision athletes. Pagnani et al. [45] looked at 58 American football players who underwent open stabilization and found no postoperative dislocations at an average follow up of 37 months and an average age of 18.2 years. Studies in the late 1990s and early 2000s, however, began to show arthroscopic stabilization results similar to open standards [46, 47]. Authors argued that patient selection according to correct identification of lesion type and tissue quality was of absolute importance in successful arthroscopic treatment. Others argued that several arthroscopic failures that were in the literature were due to nonanatomic surgical correction. They proposed that if the anterior labrum is stabilized to the anterior glenoid rim and the integrity of the IGHL is restored, the failure rates for arthroscopic stabilization would be much lower [5]. Larrain et al. [41] evaluated 204 rugby players that underwent either arthroscopic or open stabilization. This decision was based on type of Bankart lesion, tissue quality, and presence of bony defects. Of the 160 patients that underwent arthroscopic stabilization, 39 had surgery for acute instability and 121 had surgery for recurrent instability. They reported good or excellent results in 94.8 % of the acute instability group, and in 91.6 % of the recurrent instability group. Patients were selected for open stabilization if they had humeral deficiencies greater than one forth of the articular humeral head, bony glenoid deficiencies of >25 %, capsular laxity with poor tissue quality, and humeral avulsion of the glenohumeral ligament. This suggests that with appropriate patient selection, arthroscopic stabilization is an acceptable method of stabilization in collision athletes. The improvement in results over the years is likely due to the development of new implants and instrumentation, greater surgeon experience, and increased comfort with arthroscopy [2].

Arthroscopic stabilization (Figs. 2.2, 2.3, 2.4) also avoids violating the subscapularis and is associated with less loss of external rotation, making it a more attractive option in athletes [48]. Although maintenance of external rotation is more important for overhead athletes than collision athletes, it is an important consideration when deciding management.

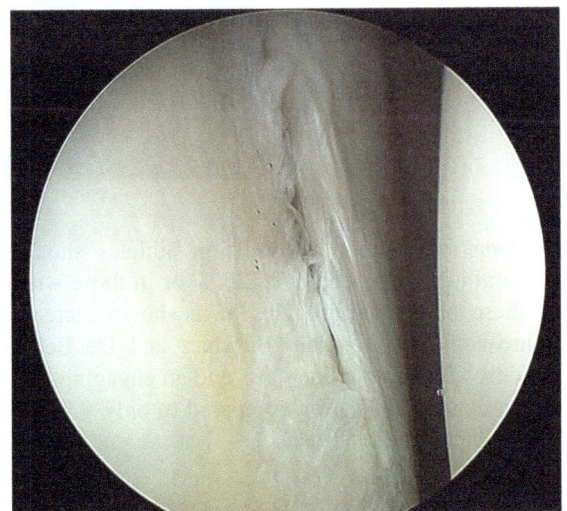

Fig. 2.2 Anterior labral tear viewed through a posterior arthroscopic portal

Fig. 2.3 Anterior labral tear viewed through a posterior arthroscopic portal

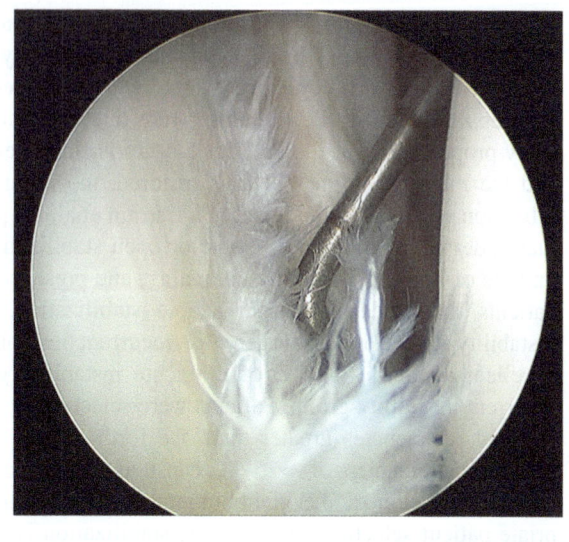

Fig. 2.4 Anterior labral repair viewed through a posterior arthroscopic portal

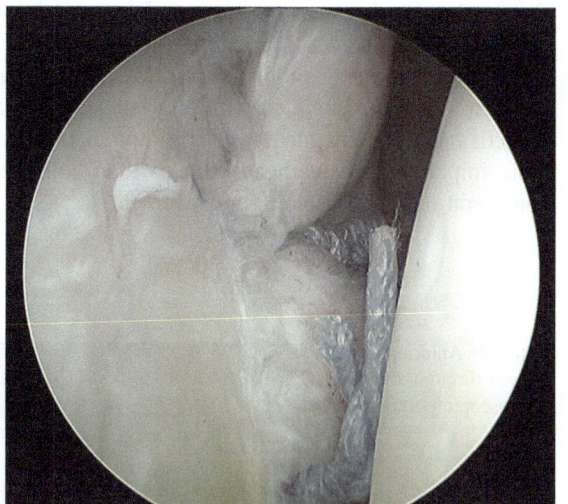

Open stabilization in collision athletes should be reserved for those with humeral head deficiency of >25 % or in those with glenoid deficiency of >25 %, as these bony morphologies have shown increased recurrence rates following arthroscopic stabilization. Burkhart and De Beer found the recurrence rate in patients with glenoid bone loss and an engaging Hill-Sachs lesion to be 67 % after arthroscopic stabilization compared to only 4 % in patients with not bony defects [24]. (Please see references [1–3] at the end of the chapter.)

References

1. Wang RY, Arciero RA (2008) Treating the athlete with anterior shoulder instability. Clin Sports Med 27:631–648
2. Owens BD, Duffey ML, Nelson BJ et al (2007) The incidence and characteristics of shoulder instability at the United States Military Academy. Am J Sports Med 35(7):1168–1173
3. Cole BJ, Warner JP (2000) Arthroscopic versus open Bankart repair for traumatic anterior shoulder instability. Clin Sports Med 19:19–48
4. Hulstyn MJ, Fadale PD (1997) Shoulder injuries in the athlete. Clin Sports Med 16:663–679
5. Lazarus MD, Harryman DT (2000) Complications of open anterior stabilization of the shoulder. J Am Acad Orthop Surg 8:122–132
6. Visser CP, Coene LN, Brand R et al (1999) The incidence of nerve injury in anterior dislocation of the shoulder and its influence on functional recovery. A prospective clinical and EMG study. J Bone Joint Surg [Br] 81-B:679–685
7. Piasecki DP, Verma NN, Romeo AA et al (2009) Glenoid bone deficiency in recurrent anterior shoulder instability: diagnosis and management. J Am Acad Orthop Surg 17:482–493
8. Gaskill TR, Taylor DC, Millett PJ (2011) Management of multidirectional instability of the shoulder. J Am Acad Orthop Surg 19:758–767
9. Kvitne RL, Jobe FW, Jobe CM (1995) Shoulder instability in the overhand or throwing athlete. Clin Sports Med 14(4):917–935
10. Skendzel JG, Sekiya JK (2012) Diagnosis and management of humeral head bone loss in shoulder instability. Am J Sports Med 40:2633–2644
11. Mologne TS, Provencher MT, Menzel KA et al (2007) Arthroscopic stabilization in patients with an inverted pear glenoid: results in patients with bone loss of the anterior glenoid. Am J Sports Med 35:1276–1283
12. Jobe FW, Kvitne RS, Giangarra CE (1989) Shoulder pain in the overhand or throwing athlete: the relationship of anterior instability and rotator cuff impingement. Ortho Rev 18(9):963–975
13. Lo IK, Nonweiler B, Woolfrey M et al (2004) An evaluation of the apprehension, relocation, and surprise tests for anterior shoulder instability. Am J Sports Med 32(2):301–307
14. Millett PJ, Clavert P, Hatch GF et al (2006) Recurrent posterior shoulder instability. J Am Acad Orthop Surg 14:464–476
15. Blasier R, Soslowsky L, Malicky D et al (1997) Posterior glenohumeral subluxation: active and passive stabilization in a biomechanical model. J Bone Joint Surg Am 79(3):433–440
16. Provencher MT, LeClere LE, King S et al (2011) Posterior instability of the shoulder: diagnosis and management. Am J Sports Med 39:874–886
17. Kim SH, Park JS, Jeong WK et al (2005) The Kim test: a novel test for posteroinferior labral lesion of the shoulder—a comparison to the jerk test. Am J Sports Med 33(8):1188–1192
18. Tzannes A, Murrell GA (2002) Clinical examination of the unstable shoulder. Sports Med 32(7):447–457
19. Edwards TB, Boulahia A, Walch G (2003) Radiographic analysis of bone defects in chronic anterior shoulder instability. Arthroscopy 19:732–739
20. Garth WP, Slappey CE, Ochs CW (1984) Roentgenographic demonstration of instability of the shoulder: the apical oblique projection—a technical note. J Bone Joint Surg Am 66:1450–1453
21. Pavlov H, Warren RF, Weiss CB et al (1985) The roentgenographic evaluation of anterior shoulder instability. Clin Orthop Relat Res 194:153–158
22. Itoi E, Lee SB, Amrami KK et al (2003) Quantitative assessment of classic anteroinferior bony Bankart lesions by radiography and computed tomography. Am J Sports Med 31:112–118
23. Sugaya H, Moriishi J, Dohi M et al (2003) Glenoid rim morphology in recurrent anterior glenohumeral instability. J Bone Joint Surg Am 85:878–884

24. Burkhart SS, De Beer JF (2000) Traumatic glenohumeral bone defects and their relationship to failure of arthroscopic Bankart repairs: significance of the inverted pear glenoid and the humeral engaging Hill-Sachs lesion. Arthroscopy 16:677–694

25. Kirkley A, Werstine R, Ratjek A et al (2005) Prospective randomized clinical trial comparing the effectiveness of immediate arthroscopic stabilization versus immobilization and rehabilitation in first traumatic anterior dislocations of the shoulder: long-term evaluation. Arthroscopy 21(1):55–63

26. Buss DD, Lynch GP, Meyer CP et al (2004) Nonoperative management for in-season athletes with anterior shoulder instability. Am J Sports Med 32(6):1430–1433

27. Robinson CM, Howes J, Murdoch H et al (2006) Functional outcome and risk of recurrent instability after primary traumatic anterior shoulder dislocation in young patients. J Bone Joint Surg Am 88(11):2326–2336

28. Burns TC, Owens BD (2010) Management of shoulder instability in in-season athletes. Phys Sports Med 38(3):55–60

29. Itoi E, Sashi R, Minagawa H et al (2001) Position of immobilization after dislocation of the glenohumeral joint: a study with use of magnetic resonance imaging. J Bone Joint Surg Am 83(5):661–667

30. Itoi E, Hatakeyama Y, Sato T et al (2007) Immobilization in external rotation after shoulder dislocation reduces risk of recurrence: a randomized controlled trial. J Bone Joint Surg Am 89(10):2124–2131

31. Liavaag S, Brox JI, Pripp AH et al (2011) Immobilization in external rotation after primary shoulder dislocation did not reduce the risk of recurrence: a randomized controlled trial. J Bone Joint Surg Am 93(10):897–904

32. Hovelius L, Eriksson K, Fredin H et al (1983) Recurrences after initial dislocation of the shoulder: results of a prospective study of treatment. J Bone Joint Surg Am 65(3):343–349

33. Aronen JG, Regan K (1984) Decreasing the incidence of recurrence of first time anterior shoulder dislocations with rehabilitation. Am J Sports Med 12(4):283–291

34. O'Brien SJ, Neves MC, Arnoczky SP et al (1990) The anatomy and histology of the inferior glenohumeral ligament of the shoulder. Am J Sports Med 18:449–456

35. Thomas SC, Matsen FA (1989) An approach to repair of avulsion of the glenohumeral ligaments in the management of traumatic anterior glenohumeral instability. J Bone Joint Surg Am 71:506–513

36. Arciero RA, Wheeler JH, Ryan JB et al (1994) Arthroscopic Bankart repair versus nonoperative treatment for acute, initial anterior shoulder dislocations. Am J Sports Med 22(5):589–594

37. Bottoni CR, Wilckens JH, DeBerardino TM et al (2002) A prospective, randomized evaluation of arthroscopic stabilization versus nonoperative treatment in patients with acute, traumatic, first time shoulder dislocations. Am J Sports Med 30(4):576–580

38. Yiannakopoulos CK, Mataragas E, Antonogiannakis E (2007) A comparison of the spectrum of intra-articular lesions in acute and chronic anterior shoulder instability. Arthroscopy 23(9):985–990

39. Urayama M, Itoi E, Sashi R et al (2003) Capsular elongation in shoulders with recurrent anterior dislocation: Quantitative assessment with magnetic resonance arthrography. Am J Sports Med 31(1):64–67

40. Taylor DC, Arciero RA (1997) Pathologic changes associated with shoulder dislocations: arthroscopic and physical examination findings in first-time, traumatic anterior shoulder dislocations. Am J Sports Med 25(3):306–311

41. Larrain MV, Montenegro HJ, Mauas DM et al (2006) Arthroscopic management of traumatic anterior shoulder instability in collision athletes: analysis of 204 cases with a 4- to 9- year follow-up and results with suture anchor technique. Arthroscopy 22(12):1283–1289

42. Cole BJ, L'Insalata J, Irrgang J et al (2000) Comparison of arthroscopic and open anterior shoulder stabilization. A two to six-year follow-up study. J Bone Joint Surg Am 82:1108–1114

43. O'Neill DB (1999) Arthroscopic Bankart repair of anterior detachments of the glenoid labrum—a prospective study. J Bone Joint Surg Am 81:1357–1366

44. Pagnani MJ, Warren RF, Altchek DW et al (1996) Arthroscopic shoulder stabilization using transglenoid sutures. A four-year minimum followup. Am J Sports Med 24:459–467

45. Pagnani MJ, Dome DC (2002) Surgical treatment of traumatic anterior shoulder instability in American football players. J Bone Joint Surg 84-A:711–715

46. Ide J, Maeda S, Takagi K (2004) Arthroscopic Bankart repair using suture anchors in athletes: patient selection and postoperative sports activity. Am J Sports Med 32:1899–1905

47. Mazzocca AD, Brown FM, Carreira DS et al (2005) Arthroscopic anterior shoulder stabilization of collision and contact athletes. Am J Sports Med 33:52–60

48. Gill TJ, Micheli LJ, Gebhard F et al (1997) Bankart repair for anterior instability of the shoulder: long-term outcome. J Bone Joint Surg Am 79(6):850–857

Arthroscopic Bony Bankart Repair/Stabilization

3

Hiroyuki Sugaya

3.1 Introduction

Glenoid anterior rim fractures, accompanied by acute glenohumeral dislocation and subluxation with tremendous amount of external force [1], usually result in persistent instability of the glenohumeral joint [2]. According to a three-dimensionally reconstructed computed tomography (3DCT) study, the prevalence of anterior glenoid bony lesion has been reported as high as 90 % in shoulders with chronic recurrent traumatic anterior instability and an associated bony fragment is present in about a half of shoulders with anterior glenoid bony lesion [3]. Further, bone loss in shoulders associated with a bony fragment is relatively significant compared to that in shoulders with attritional glenoid without bony fragment [3, 4].

In shoulders with bony Bankart lesion, a bone fragment is firmly connected to the labrum because the majority of the anterior glenoid rim fractures are avulsion type glenoid rim fracture [4–6]. In acute cases, it is widely accepted that such glenoid fractures with a large fragment [7], and/or displacement of more than 10 mm [8], and associated instability [2], immediate surgical fragment reduction and fixation using screws [7] or suture anchors [6, 9, 10] is indicated either open or arthroscopically. On the other hand, in chronic shoulders with recurrent instability, surgeons need to respect entire glenohumeral ligament pathology, such as capsular lesions or elongation of the capsule, in addition to the bone loss [11]. Glenoid bone loss is relatively significant when a bony fragment is present [3, 4]. In addition, some authors reported excellent surgical outcomes after arthroscopic fragment fixation along with capsulolabral reconstruction [4, 10, 12, 13]. However, many surgeons tend to ignore the fragment, partly because they do not believe that the

H. Sugaya (✉)
Shoulder & Elbow Service, Funabashi Orthopaedic Sports Medicine Center,
1-833 Hasama, Funabashi, Chiba 2740822, Japan
e-mail: hsugaya@nifty.com

S. F. Brockmeier et al. (eds.), *Surgery of Shoulder Instability*,
DOI: 10.1007/978-3-642-38100-3_3, © ISAKOS 2013

bony fragment associated with chronic shoulder instability is viable in addition to possible complexity of the procedure, and prefer to perform the coracoid transfer [14, 15] which is simple but relatively invasive and non-anatomical procedure. In the meantime, Fujii and colleagues proved that these bony fragments are viable even in chronic lesion because their blood supply to the bone fragment was maintained through the adjacent soft tissue [16]. Therefore, these shoulders are favorable candidates for arthroscopic bony Bankart repair associate with capsular tensioning of the entire glenohumeral ligament [4, 5, 17, 18]. Many shoulders associated with bony Bankart lesion can be reparable because small to medium size fragment can be easily incorporated to the Bankart repair without excising the bony fragment. However, it is true that there exist difficult cases in shoulders associated with medium to large bony fragment because surgeons need to stabilize the fragment by passing through or around it. We have developed a very handy device for managing these large fragments. In this article, updated version of technical pearls for arthroscopic bony Bankart repair is described in detail.

3.2   Diagnosis

The diagnosis of recurrent traumatic anterior glenohumeral instability is usually made easily on the basis of the history of distinct dislocation or subluxation and the positive apprehension sign. The anterior apprehension test is done with the patient in the supine position. In this test, the shoulder is moved passively into maximum external rotation with the arm at side, 30, 60, 90, 120, 150° of abduction, and maximum flexion [17, 18]. At the same time, the posterior apprehension test is done with the arm at maximum internal rotation in 90° of abduction. The feeling of apprehension is reported in each arm position. However, the most important and reliable physical examination can usually be done with the patient under anesthesia, comparing stability testing to the contralateral shoulder.

3.3   Imaging

X-ray images are sometimes helpful in detecting the Hill-Sachs lesion and the anterior glenoid rim lesion, especially during the first patient visit. Bernageau described an effective method for detecting an anterior glenoid rim lesion with the patients in the standing position [19]. However, this technique requires fluoroscopic control in order to obtain optimal diagnosable images and, therefore, radiation exposure is an unignorable issue [20]. We have developed a modified Bernageau method with the patient lying on their axilla in their most relaxed position [17, 18]. In this method, clear X-ray images can be obtained more easily with a high probability of ascertaining bony pathology without using fluoroscopic imaging [17, 18].

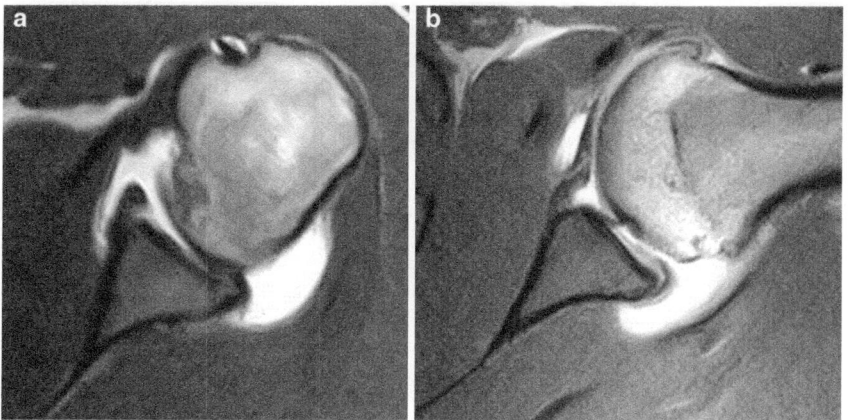

Fig. 3.1 MR arthrography in the shoulder with a bony Bankart lesion. **a** Axial view, **b** ABER (abduction and external rotation) view. Although only Bankart lesion is detectable in the axial view, slack IGHL and the humeral head translation in addition to the Bankart lesion is detectable in the ABER view

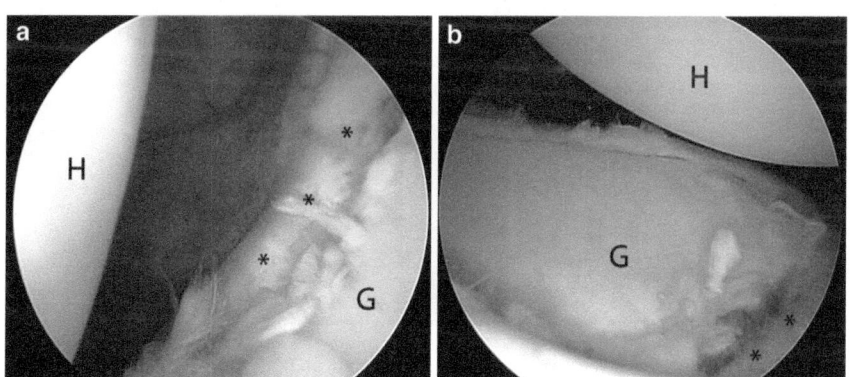

Fig. 3.2 Arthroscopic view of the same shoulder as Fig. 3.1. **a** A view from the posterior portal. **b** A view from the anterior portal. *H* humeral head, *G* glenoid, *Asterisks* indicate bony fragment embedded in the surrounding soft tissue

Plain MRI provides only limited information for shoulder instability. However, MR-Arthrography is helpful when detecting a soft tissue lesion such as a Bankart lesion, capsular pathology, and/or a HAGL (humeral avulsion of the glenohumeral ligament) lesion (Fig. 3.1). Nonetheless, the final diagnosis of soft tissue pathology can be made most accurately through diagnostic arthroscopy (Fig. 3.2).

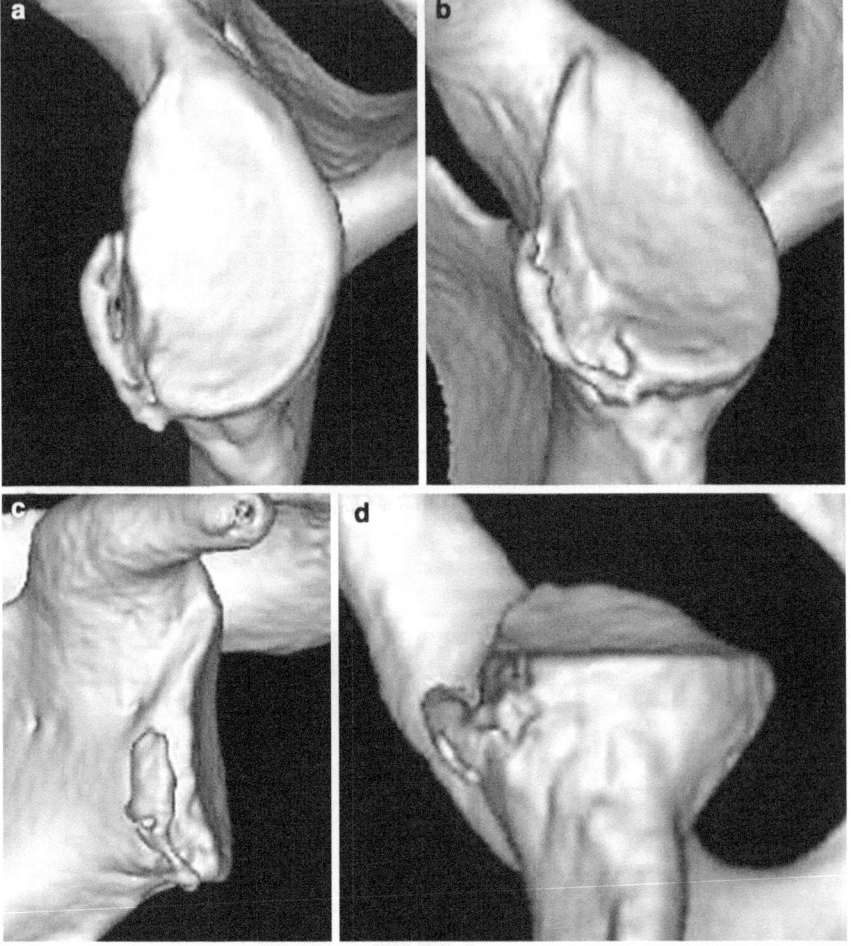

Fig. 3.3 3DCT images of the same shoulder as Figs. 3.1 and 3.2. Surgeons need to recognize size and shape of the bone fragment prior to surgery in order to manage the fragment during surgery. **a** En face view, **b** oblique view, **c** anterior view, **d** inferior view

3DCT is the most important imaging study in order to assess glenoid morphology accurately [3]. In a shoulder with bony Bankart lesion, detecting accurate configuration of the bony fragment during surgery is not easy because the bone fragment is covered by the surrounding soft tissue. Through preoperative 3DCT, surgeons can assess the size and shape of the bony fragment in shoulders with a bony Bankart lesion (Fig. 3.3) [3, 4, 21].

3.4   Surgery

Regardless of the severity of glenoid bone loss, arthroscopic bony Bankart repair is indicated if an apparent bone fragment is present with 3DCT [4, 5]. Since the majority of shoulders with a large glenoid bone loss retains bony fragment at the anteroinferior glenoid neck [17, 18], this procedure is applicable to most shoulders with significant glenoid bone loss. Normally, in shoulders with bony Bankart lesion, the fragment is medially displaced and partly united to the glenoid neck, and also the fragment is firmly connected to the adjacent labrum or soft tissue (Figs. 3.2, 3.3, 3.4a). Therefore, the bony fragment associated with a bony Bankart

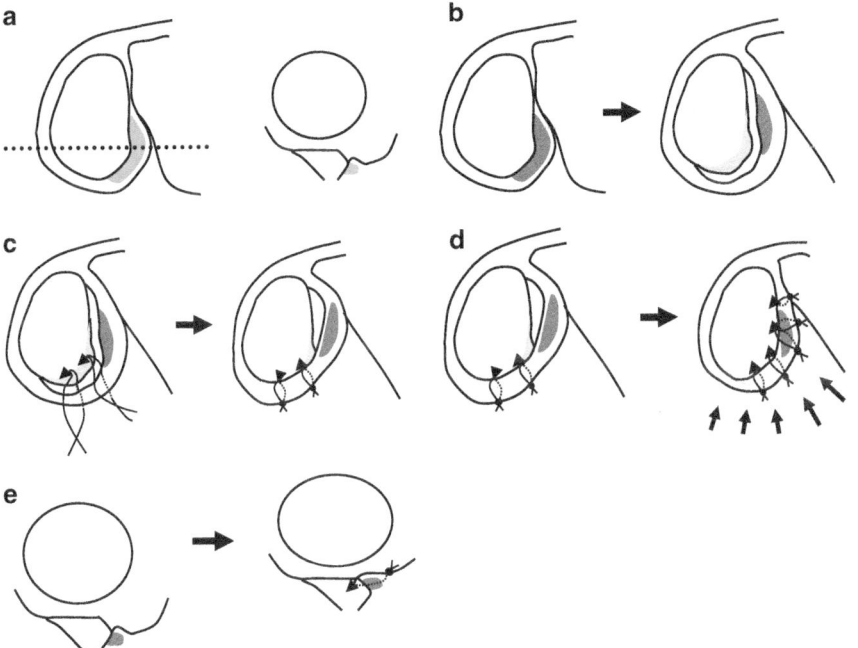

Fig. 3.4 Schematic drawings of entire surgical procedures. In shoulders with bony Bankart lesion, the fragment is normally medially displaced and partly united to the glenoid neck, and also the fragment is firmly connected to the adjacent labrum or soft tissue. The *dotted line* indicates the plane of the axial section (**a**). After separation of the fragment and labrum from the glenoid neck, the mobilization of the labroligamentous complex is performed up to the 7:30 position in the right shoulder until the complex and the fragment become completely free. In addition, articular cartilage on the edge of the glenoid is also removed (**b**). Then, two suture anchors are inserted to the face of the inferior glenoid and the inferior labrum was first reduced. Thanks to this procedure, the bony fragment was automatically brought upward and, therefore, handling of the fragment becomes easier (**c**). Next, bony fragment is stabilized by pulling the adjacent labrum with a grasper inserted through the anterosuperior portal. Then, a bone penetrating instrument is inserted though the anterior portal and sutures are placed to the fragment. Knot tying provides not just fragment reduction but proper tensioning to the entire inferior glenohumeral ligament (**d, e**). The *gray* area on the glenoid indicates the area where articular cartilage is removed. The *dark* area on the labrum side indicates a bony fragment inside the soft tissue

lesion can be easily separated from the glenoid neck using standard straight or curved rasps. Although the gap between the fragment and original glenoid is well demarcated in most shoulders, if otherwise, careful palpation or preoperative 3DCT greatly help surgeons to delineate the gap (Fig. 3.3) [17, 18].

3.4.1 Patient Positioning and EUA

All patients are seated in the beach-chair position under general anesthesia and/or interscalene block and joint laxity is assessed by examination of both shoulders prior to surgical intervention. General anesthesia is preferable because surgeons can assess constitutional laxity on the contralateral side during EUA.

3.4.2 Portals and Diagnostic Arthroscopy

A 4 mm arthroscope is introduced through a standard posterior portal and a diagnostic arthroscopy is performed. Then an anterior portal is created just superior to the subscapularis tendon and just lateral to the conjoined tendon using an outside-in technique, in order to facilitate instrument insertion without cannulas [22]. Then, arthroscope is switched to the anterior portal and diagnostic arthroscopy is performed in order to evaluate capsular integrity and confirm a bony Bankart lesion (Fig. 3.2). In addition, an anterosuperior portal is established at the anterosuperior margin of the rotator interval utilizing an outside-in technique. This becomes the second working portal. In shoulders with superior labral detachment, a lateral acromial portal, established just lateral to the mid-point of the acromion through the muscle–tendon junction of the infraspinatus, is used instead of the anterosuperior portal (Fig. 3.5).

3.4.3 Surgical Procedures

3.4.3.1 Mobilization of the Complex
After diagnostic arthroscopy from the anterior portal, arthroscope is again switched to the posterior portal. Then, separation and mobilization of the labroligamentous complex together with the bony fragment from the glenoid neck is performed using an elevator, straight and curved rasps, scissors, shavers, and a radiofrequency probe. All of these instrument tools are inserted through a cannulaless anterior portal. This step is a vital part of this procedure.

First, a straight rasp is inserted from the anterior portal and is placed in the small gap between the fragment and the glenoid neck. Then, the gap is expanded by tapping the handle of the rasp (Fig. 3.6a). After separating the fragment from the glenoid neck, the mobilization of the labroligamentous complex is performed up to the 7:30 position in the right shoulder until the complex and the fragment

Fig. 3.5 Portal placement. A drawing demonstrates the right shoulder seen from above. In addition to standard posterior and anterior rotator interval portal, the anterosuperior portal is used for Bankart repair. Shoulders associated with type V SLAP lesion, the lateral acromial portal is used instead of the anterosuperior portal

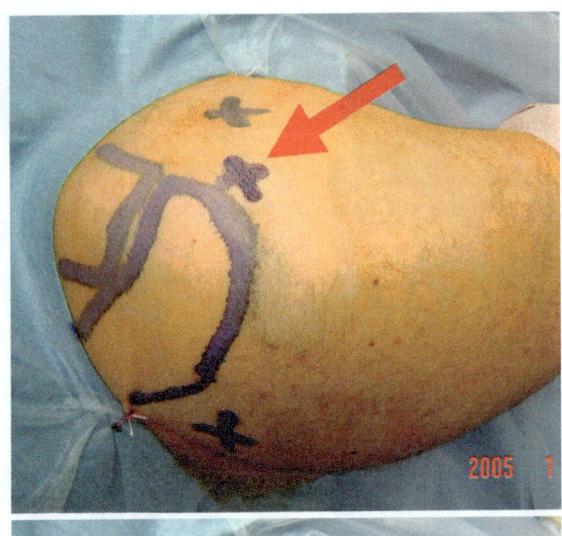

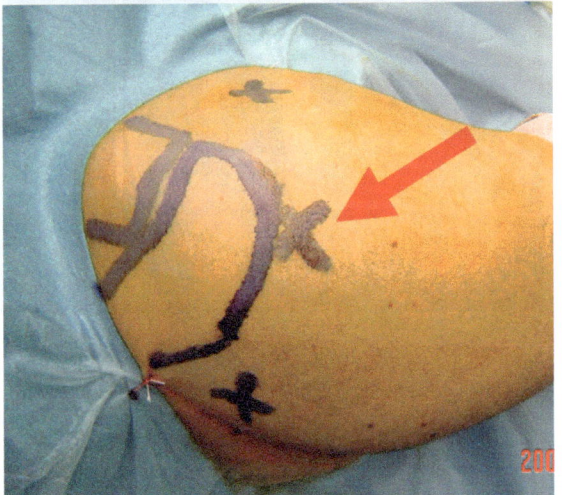

become completely free in exactly the same way as one would mobilize a Bankart lesion without a bone fragment using the instruments previously described. Further, articular cartilage on the edge of the glenoid is also removed to promote tissue healing after repair (Figs. 3.4b and 3.6b). Normally, the separation of the fragment from the neck can be readily accomplished using only elevators and rasps. If the separation of the fragment is difficult and the fragment is united firmly, a small size chisel can be introduced from the anterior portal to separate it from the glenoid neck.

Pearls: Recognize the size, shape, and location of the bony fragment using preoperative 3DCT prior to surgery (Fig. 3.3).

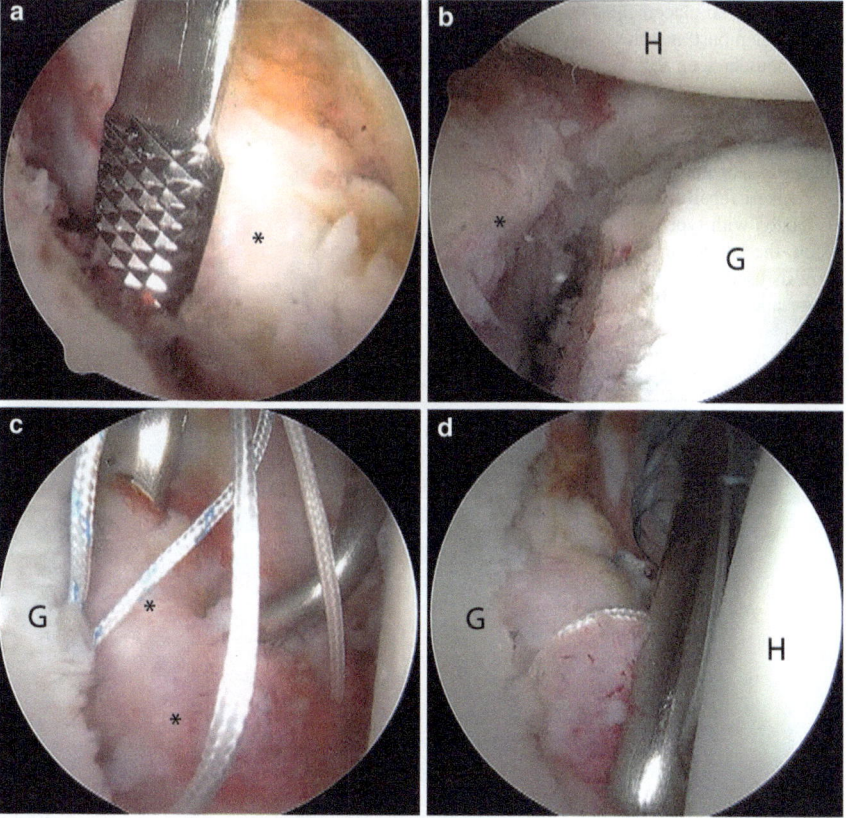

Fig. 3.6 Surgical procedures. A bony fragment and adjacent labrum is separated from the glenoid neck using a rasp (**a**). Arthroscopic view after complete separation and mobilization of the complex, viewing from the anterior portal. Articular cartilage at the margin of the inferior glenoid face was removed (**b**). A grasper inserted through the anterosuperior portal stabilizes the bony fragment by pulling the adjacent labrum and a bone penetrating instrument inserted though the anterior portal is trying to penetrate the fragment through the surrounding soft tissue (**c**). Knot tying after suture placement to the fragment (**d**). The *asterisk* indicates the bony fragment embedded in the surrounding soft tissue. *H* humeral head, *G* glenoid

3.4.3.2 Repair of Inferior Labrum Adjacent to the Osseous Fragment

The following procedure is very important in order to obtain optimal fragment reduction and provide proper tension to the inferior glenohumeral ligament. The following procedure is performed using the posterior portal as a viewing portal, and the anterior and anterosuperior portal as working portals.

The first suture anchor loaded with #2 high strength suture is inserted on the surface of the glenoid at the 6 o'clock position using a drill guide introduced through the cannulaless anterior portal. Because this portal has no cannula, the angle of approach of the guide can be adjusted easily allowing optimization of the angle to the glenoid [22]. After the first anchor insertion, a looped #2-0 nylon suture is placed into the labrum at the 6:30 position using a low profile 7 mm Caspari Punch™ (Conmed Linvatec, Largo, FL, USA) or a Suture Hook™ (Conmed Linvatec, Largo, FL, USA). A suture relay is then performed intra-articularly [22]. The second anchor is inserted into the face of the glenoid at the 4:40 position, followed by the suture placement in the labrum adjacent to the inferior side of the bony fragment using the same technique (Fig. 3.4c). After completion of the suture placement of the inferior two anchors, knot tying is performed using a self-locking sliding knot through a cannula inserted through the anterior portal. To accomplish secure knot tying, the complex, together with the fragment, is held upward and laterally on the glenoid surface by a grasper introduced through the anterosuperior portal to reduce tensile force on the suture.

3.4.3.3 Osseous Fragment and Superior Labrum Repair

The next step is the suturing of the osseous fragment itself, either by passing the suture through the fragment or by penetrating it using bone penetrating tools such as a Bone Stitcher™ (Smith and Nephew, Andover, MA, USA), which is an originally developed bone penetrator with a stiff shaft and large handle (Fig. 3.7), or by passing suture around the fragment using a Suture Hook™ or Suture Leader™ (Depuy Mitek, Raynham, MA, USA) and/or Bone Stitcher™ [5, 17, 18]. It is very important to characterize the fragment shape and size preoperatively by 3DCT evaluation to decide whether passing through or passing around the fragment is most appropriate (Fig. 3.3) [5, 17, 18]. This procedure is facilitated when the bony fragment is reduced and stabilized by grasping cranial portion of the labrum adjacent to the fragment with a grasper introduced from the anterosuperior portal (Fig. 3.6c). Although the number of suture anchors utilized is dependent on the size and shape of the osseous fragment, normally one or two suture anchors are used for stabilizing the bony fragment [5, 17, 18]. Knot tying is performed after placing the sutures through the fragment (Figs. 3.4d and 3.6d). The final step is to suture the labrum adjacent to the cranial side of fragment to augment the stability of the entire complex. Normally four suture anchors with simple sutures are used to reconstruct the entire labroligamentous complex (Figs. 3.4e and 3.8).

Pearls: During above procedure, the arthroscope need to stay in the posterior portal and both the anterior and anterosuperior portals are used as working portals. A 30° scope is enough but a 70° scope may be helpful. In order to penetrate the medium to large bony fragment nicely, surgeons need to reduce and stabilize a bony fragment by grasping the cranial side of the labrum adjacent to the fragment

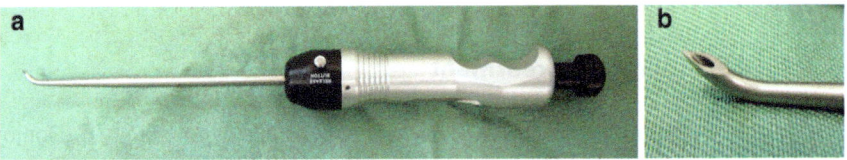

Fig. 3.7 Bone Stitcher™ (Smith and Nephew, Andover, MA)

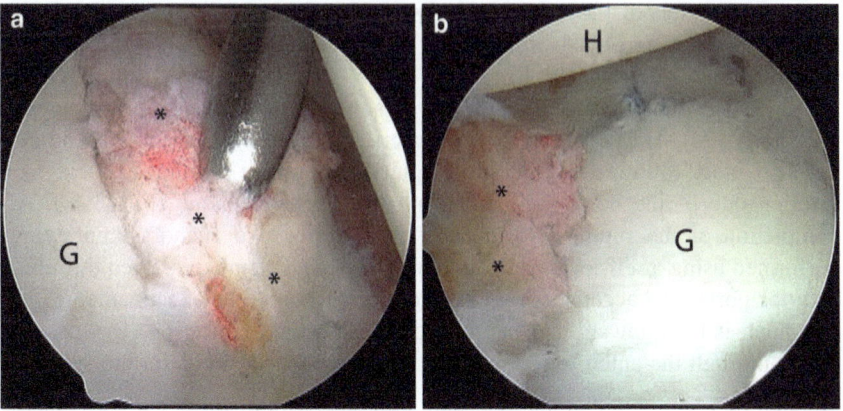

Fig. 3.8 Arthroscopic appearance after completing bony Bankart repair, viewing from the posterior portal (**a**), and the anterior portal (**b**). The *asterisk* indicates the bony fragment embedded in the surrounding soft tissue. *H* humeral head, *G* glenoid

with a grasper introduced from the anterosuperior portal. Then, aim the blade of the Bone Stitcher perpendicular to the fragment. After catching the bony fragment by the tip of the Bone Stitcher, push the fragment to the neck of the glenoid and then penetrate it by rotating the blade of the Bone Stitcher applying a force perpendicular to the glenoid neck.

3.4.3.4 Management of the Associated Pathology

In shoulders with a capsular tear, a capsular repair utilizing two to three side-to-side stitches is performed prior to the bony Bankart repair. Furthermore, in shoulders with a superior labral detachment, arthroscopic reattachment is performed, after the Bony Bankart repair is completed, utilizing a lateral acromial portal instead of the anterosuperior portal (Fig. 3.5).

3.4.3.5 Augmentation

The rotator interval closure and/or Hill-Sachs Remplissage [23] is performed as an augmentation in patients with relatively high-risk shoulders, such as contact athletes, young and lax individuals, and those with a large Hill-Sachs lesion. In those patients, the rotator interval is closed by suturing the superior margin of the subscapularis tendon to the superior glenohumeral ligament with the arm held at the side and in maximum external rotation using #2 high strength sutures [17, 18, 24].

3.4.4 Postoperative Treatment

The shoulders are immobilized for 3 weeks using a sling (Ultra Sling III, Donjoy, Carlsbad, CA). After immobilization, passive and assisted-active exercises are initiated for forward flexion and external rotation avoiding pain. After 6 weeks, patients begin strengthening exercises of the rotator cuff and scapular stabilizers. Three months after the operation, they are permitted to practice non-contact sports. Full return to throwing or contact sports is allowed after 6 months according to each individual's functional recovery. Excessive mechanical stress to the reconstructed site within 3 months after surgery may cause anchor/suture failure. In order to avoid this, instruct patients not to be too active until 3 months after surgery.

3.5 Summary

Prevalence of a bony Bankart lesion is very high especially collision/contact athletes in recurrent anterior glenohumeral instability and the most of shoulders with large glenoid defect retains a bony fragment at the anteroinferior glenoid neck [17, 18]. In addition, since a bony Bankart lesion is an avulsion type glenoid rim fracture, normally the fragment and labrum junction is intact even in a chronic case. Therefore, although sometimes technically demanding in shoulders with large fragment, arthroscopic bony Bankart repair is technically feasible regardless of fragment or glenoid defect size. If surgeons can understand every single pearls of the entire procedure described in this article, I believe arthroscopic bony Bankart repair, which is less invasive and anatomical procedure, becomes easy and outcome promising surgery for every surgeons.

References

1. Aston JW, Gregory CF (1973) Dislocation of the shoulder with significant fracture of the glenoid. J Bone Joint Surg Am 55:1531–1533
2. Ideberg R (1984) Fractures of the scapula involving the glenoid fossa. In: Bateman JE, Welsh RP (eds) Surgery of the shoulder. BC Decker, Toronto, pp 63–66
3. Sugaya H, Moriishi J, Dohi M, Kon Y, Tsuchiya A (2003) Glenoid rim morphology in recurrent anterior glenohumeral instability. J Bone Joint Surg Am 85:878–884
4. Sugaya H, Moriishi J, Kanisawa I, Tsuchiya A (2005) Arthroscopic osseous Bankart repair for chronic recurrent traumatic anterior glenohumeral instability. J Bone Joint Surg Am 87A:1752–1760
5. Sugaya H, Moriishi J, Kanisawa I, Tsuchiya A (2006) Arthroscopic osseous Bankart repair for chronic traumatic anterior glenohumeral instability. Surgical technique. J Bone Joint Surg Am 88A(Supplement 1 part 2):159–169
6. Sugaya H, Kon Y, Tsuchiya A (2005) Arthroscopic repair of glenoid fractures using suture anchors: technical note with cases series. Arthroscopy 21:635.e1–635.e5
7. Rockwood CA, Matsen FA (1990) The scapula. In: Butters KP (ed) The shoulder. WB Saunders, Philadelphia, pp 345–353
8. De Palma AF (1983) Fractures and fracture-dislocations of the shoulder girdle. In: Jacob RP, Kristainsen T, Mayo K et al (eds) Surgery of the shoulder, 3rd edn. JB Lippincott, Philadelphia pp 366–367
9. Cameron SE (1998) Arthroscopic reduction and internal fixation of an anterior glenoid fracture. Arthroscopy 14:743–746

10. Porcellini G, Campi F, Paladini P (2002) Arthroscopic approach to acute bony Bankart lesion. Arthroscopy 18:764–769
11. Shapiro TA, Gupta A, McGarry MH, Tibone JE, Lee TQ (2012) Biomechanical effects of arthroscopic capsulorrhaphy in line with the fibers of the anterior band of the inferior glenohumeral ligament. Am J Sports Med 40:672–680
12. Park JY, Lee SJ, Lhee SH, Lee SH (2012) Follow-up computed tomography arthrographic evaluation of bony Bankart lesions after arthroscopic repair. Arthroscopy 28(4):465–473
13. Mologne TS, Provencher MT, Menzel KA, Vachon TA, Dewing CB (2007) Arthroscopic stabilization in patients with an inverted pear glenoid: results in patients with bone loss of the anterior glenoid. Am J Sports Med 35:1276–1283
14. Latarjet M (1965) Techniques chirugicales dans le trairement de la luxation anteriointerne recidivante de l'epaule. Lyon Chir 61:313–318
15. Lafosse L, Lejeune E, Bouchard A, Kakuda C, Gobezie R, Kochhar T (2007) The arthroscopic Latarjet procedure for the treatment of anterior shoulder instability. Arthroscopy 23:1242.e1–1242.e5
16. Fujii Y, Yoneda M, Wakitani S, Hayashida K (2006) Histologic analysis of bony Bankart lesions in recurrent anterior instability of the shoulder. J Should Elbow Surg 15:218–223
17. Sugaya H (2010) Chapter 14: Instability with bone loss. In: Angelo RL, Esch JC, Ryu RK (eds) AANA advanced arthroscopy: the shoulder. Elsevier, Philadelphia, pp 136–146
18. Sugaya H (2011) Section 2 anterior instability: chapter 15 arthroscopic treatment of glenoid bone loss—surgical technique. In: Provencher M, Romeo A (eds) Shoulder instability a comprehensive approach. Elsevier, Philadelphia, pp 186–196
19. Bernageau J (1990) Imaging of the shoulder in orthopedic pathology. Rev Prat Apr 40(11):983–992 (French)
20. Edwards TB, Boulahia A, Walch G (2003) Radiographic analysis of bone defects in chronic anterior shoulder instability. Arthroscopy 19:732–739
21. Chuang TY, Adams CR, Burkhart SS (2008) Use of preoperative three-dimensional computed tomography to quantify glenoid bone loss in shoulder instability. Arthroscopy 24:376–382
22. Sugaya H, Kon Y, Tsuchiya A (2004) Arthroscopic Bankart repair in the beach-chair position: a cannulaless method using intra-articular suture relay technique. Arthroscopy 20(suppl 2):116–120
23. Boileau P, O'Shea K, Vargas P, Pinedo M, Old J, Zumstein M (2012) Anatomical and functional results after arthroscopic Hill-Sachs remplissage. J Bone Joint Surg Am 94(7):618–626
24. Takahashi N, Sugaya H, Matsuki K, Tsuchiya A, Moriya H (2005) Arthroscopic rotator interval closure for recurrent anterior-inferior glenohumeral instability. Kansetsukyo (Arthroscopy) 30:57–60 (Japanese)

Latarjet/Bristow Procedure: Indications, Techniques, and Outcomes

4

Emilio Calvo and Diana Morcillo

Arthroscopic Bankart repair is regarded as the "gold standard" treatment for anterior shoulder instability. Although the results of arthroscopic anterior labral repair using modern arthroscopic techniques have been shown to approach the success rates of open anterior stabilizations in most patients [23, 29] it has been recognized that it is much less effective in patients with certain risk factors for failure such as young age, hyperlaxity, competitive contact sport participation, and especially severe glenoid or humeral bone loss [3, 6, 8]. Other techniques different to labral repair have been proposed for these patients, and coracoid transfer procedures have raised particular attention [7]. This recognition has been reinforced by recent publications [4, 25] showing the possibility of performing these complex techniques using minimally invasive and arthroscopic shoulder surgery. Once certain technical challenges are overcome the authors believe that the use of arthroscopic coracoid transfer procedures will expand among the orthopaedic community.

4.1 Coracoid Transfer Techniques

The aim of coracoid transfer techniques is to stabilise the shoulder by the static action of the transferred bone block and the dynamic action of the coracobraquialis tendon. Latarjet [27] was the first to treat anterior instability with coracoid transfer to the anterior glenoid. The Latarjet procedure involves the detachment of the pectoralis minor from the coracoid process, the incision of the coracoacromial

E. Calvo (✉) · D. Morcillo
Shoulder and Elbow Reconstructive Surgery Unit, Department of Orthopedic
Surgery and Traumatology, Fundación Jiménez Díaz—Capio, Autónoma University,
Madrid, Spain
e-mail: ecalvo@fjd.es
URL: www.fjd.es

S. F. Brockmeier et al. (eds.), *Surgery of Shoulder Instability*, 49
DOI: 10.1007/978-3-642-38100-3_4, © ISAKOS 2013

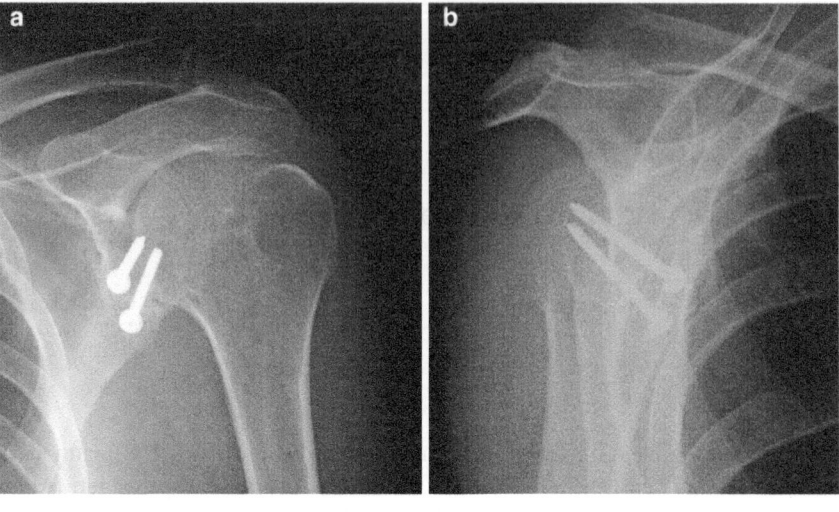

Fig. 4.1 Anteroposterior (**a**) and alar (**b**) X-Ray views of a Latarjet procedure

ligament leaving a stump of the ligament attached to the coracoid, and the completion of an osteotomy at the base of the coracoid so that it could be mobilised and placed as a bone block against the anterior glenoid neck. The coracoid process is passed through a horizontal split performed between the superior two thirds and the inferior third of the subscapularis muscle fibers, and positioned vertically adjacent to the articular surface on the inferior equator of the anterior glenoid neck, where it is secured with two screws (Figs. 4.1 and 4.2). The stabilizing effect of the technique is obtained by four mechanisms: first, the increase of the articular surface by the bone graft, second, the sling effect provided by the conjoined tendon when is tensioned in abduction and external rotation, the tensioning of the lower subscapularis by means of the conjoined tendon in its new position, and the reinforcement of the anterior ligament structures by suturing the stump of the coracoacromial ligament on the anterior capsule.

The Bristow operation was published by Helfet in 1958 [16], and consisted originally of detaching the tip of the coracoid process from the scapula just distal to the insertion of pectoralis major and leaving the conjoined tendon attached. The coracoid process with its attached tendon was transferred to a decorticated anterior surface of the glenoid neck through a vertical split in the subcapularis tendon, and fixed with a single screw. Later, Mead and Sweeney [28]. modified the technique by splitting the subscapularis muscle and tendon in line with its fibers and reported the first series of patients operated with the technique. Although Helfet reported that the procedure not only reinforced the defective part of the joint but also had a "bone block" effect, Mead and Sweeney [28] did not regard the bone block effect as being very important in stabilising the shoulder.

Fig. 4.2 Postoperative
computed tomography axial
view of an arthroscopic
Latarjet. The graft is
positioned flush with the joint
surface

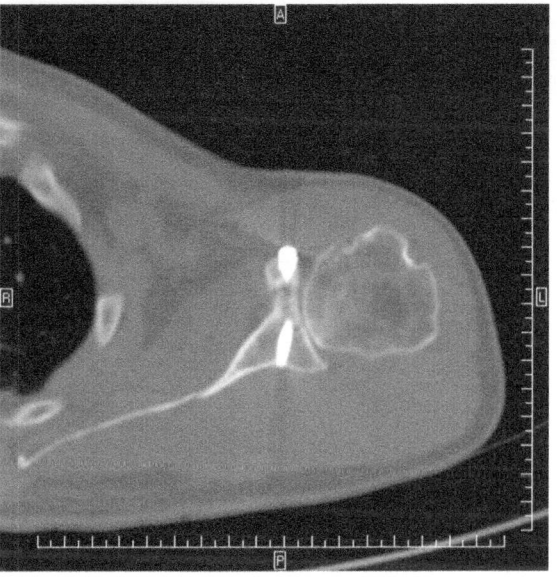

Burkhart and de Beer further modified the Latarjet technique, developing the
"congruent-arc Latarjet procedure", and designed specific instruments to position
the graft (Burkhart 2007). This technique incorporates two modifications to the
original Latarjet procedure: the coracoid graft is rotated 90° around its long axis so
that the concave inferior aspect of the coracoid becomes the extension of the
glenoid articular concavity, and the capsule is reattached to the native glenoid
using suture anchors so that the coracoid graft remains extraarticular. The ratio-
nales for these modifications are both, to obtain a more anatomic articular arc to
the reconstructed glenoid surface, and to prevent abrasion of the humeral articular
surface against the coracoid graft interposition of the glenohumeral capsule.

Lafosse et al. [25] first described the all-arthroscopic technique of the Latarjet
procedure, and developed specific tools and cannulated screws to perform it
(Fig. 4.3). On the other hand, Boileau et al. [4] reported in 2007 the "belt-and-
suspenders" arthroscopic Bristow procedure for anterior shoulder instability. An
arthroscopic Bankart repair is added to the stabilisation effect of the conjoined
tendon with this technique. The tenodesis of the conjoined tendon can be achieved
using interfragmentary screws, interference screws or suspensory fixation devices
[37]. In addition to the usual benefits of arthroscopic treatment, as lower morbidity
and faster recovery than open surgery, arthroscopic surgery in coracoid transfer
procedures provides other advantages, including the possibility of achieving a
more precise positioning of the graft, and the identification and treatment of
concomitant pathologies.

Fig. 4.3 Intraoperative view
of an arthroscopic Latarjet.
sc subscapularis, *hh* humeral
head, *cp* coracoid process,
ct conjoined tendon

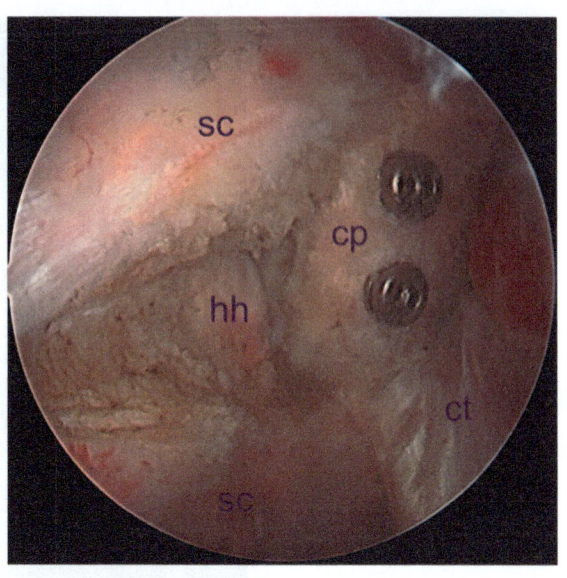

4.2   Indications for Coracoid Transfer Techniques

Coracoid transfer techniques have a long history in Europe, where they have been
regarded as the procedure of choice in anterior shoulder instability by certain
surgeons [1, 17]. However, the most frequent accepted indication for coracoid
transfer techniques is anterior shoulder instability encompassing a bony Bankart
lesion or a true fracture of the anterior or inferior glenoid rim [7]. The rationale for
this indication is to reconstruct the glenoid surface with the coracoid. There is not
clear consensus on the minimum size of the bony lesion to indicate the procedure,
but we found that glenoid loss of more than 15 % of the inferior glenoid diameter
represents a superior risk of postoperative recurrence after shoulder stabilization
with arthroscopic Bankart [8].

The presence of a large engaging Hill-Sachs lesion is considered an indication
to perform the capsulotenodesis of the posterior capsule and the infraspinatus
tendon to the humeral bone defect (remplissage) or a bone graft to the humeral
head [32]. The Latarjet technique will lengthen the arc of the anterior glenoid,
thereby increasing the degree of external rotation that can be achieved before the
lesion approaches the glenoid rim in these cases. Furthermore, a large Hill-Sachs
lesion frequently occurs in combination with glenoid bone loss. In this way, the
Latarjet operation effectively addresses both lesions without the need for additional procedure on the humeral head.

Another potential indication for coracoid transfer techniques is in the patient
with severe soft tissue loss involving the anterior labroligamentous structures.
Such deficient soft tissues can be found in patients with intrinsic poor tissue quality

or after multiple failed soft tissue procedures for instability or thermal capsular necrosis. The "sling effect" of the conjoined tendon provided by the coracoid transfer resists the anterior translation of the humeral head in the position of abduction and external rotation, but also the lengthening of the anterior glenoid arc effectively prevents glenohumeral dislocation. Although some authors have recommended using soft tissue allografts, this especial setting can also be amenable of coracoid transfer techniques based on the intraoperative observation in revision cases that a new anterior pseudocapsular tissue is formed after the Latarjet technique. Concerning other soft tissue abnormalities, Lafosse and Boyle [26] also consider the presence of a HAGL lesion an indication for shoulder stabilisation using the arthroscopic Latarjet technique based on their disappointing experience of a higher risk of shoulder stiffness after soft-tissue repair technique with anchors The group. Lyonnais conducted by Gilles Walch reported also satisfactory results of open Latarjet in cases of recurrent shoulder instability associated with rotator cuff tears [22].

Gerber and coworkers (2012) have recently shown that coracoid transfer as described by Latarjet can effectively restore anterior glenohumeral shoulder stability if previous operation(s) have failed to do so. Our preliminary experience with arthroscopic Latarjet on patients undergoing anterior shoulder instability revision surgery has been also satisfactory [9]. This applies predominantly for patients with bone defects or poor anterior sift tissue quality, but also in a specific group in whom the Bankart repair appeared successfully healed, and there is not apparent reason for the recurrence.

Patients engaged in high-risk sports (climbing, rugby, football) or occupations needing a safe and stable shoulder, or who have a high risk of recurrence due to the intensity and action of their activity are also ideal candidates for these procedures [10, 30].

It is well known that epilepsy can be devastating for shoulder stability [15]. Shoulder instability in epileptic patients is frequently associated with large bone defects and poor outcome. Coracoid transfer techniques may offer a stronger reconstruction than soft tissue procedures in these patients.

4.3 Outcomes of Coracoid Transfer Techniques

The reported outcomes of coracoid transfer techniques for anterior shoulder instability have been satisfactory, with good and consistent objective results and high degree of patient satisfaction. Hovelius et al. have reported in several papers from 1983 to 2011 the results after a long-term follow up of a homogeneous cohort patients treated with the Bristow operation for anterior shoulder instability [17–21]. In the longest follow-up study of 319 shoulders the authors report a 5 % redislocation, and a 13 % subluxation rate respectively. Three shoulders (1 %) underwent revision surgery because of remaining instability [21]. Radiographs showed bony healing in 246 of 297 shoulders (83 %), fibrous union in 34 (13 %), migration by 0.5 cm or more in 14 (5 %), and no visualization in 3 (1 %). The authors found a statistical correlation between the placement of the graft medial to the glenoid rim and the rate of recurrence, and recommended adding a horizontal capsular shift to the coracoid transfer.

Torg and co-workers [38] reported their experience with 212 modified Bristow procedures. In their modification the coracoid was passed over the superior border rather than through of the subscapularis. Their postoperative instability rate was 8,5 % (3,8 % redislocation and 4,7 % subluxation). Ten patients required reoperation for screw-related problems, 34 % had residual shoulder pain, 8 % were unable to do overhead work and only 16 % of athletes were able to return to their preinjury level of throwing. Wredmark and colleagues [39] found only 2 of 44 recurrent dislocations at an average follow–up of 6 years, but 38 % of patients complained of pain. Banas and associates [2] reported a 4 % recurrence rate with an 8,6 year follow-up; however additional surgery was required in 14 %. The modified Bristow procedure was the procedure of choice for anterior shoulder instability among midshipmen at the United States Naval Academy in the seventies. Schroeder and coworkers [35] reported the results of the modified Bristow procedure in 52 shoulders in 49 midshipmen reviewed at a mean follow-up of 26.4 years. The authors found nearly 70 % good and excellent results. Recurrent instability occurred in 8 of 52 shoulders (15.4 %), with recurrent dislocation in 5 shoulders (9.6 %) and recurrent subluxation in 3 shoulders (5.8 %).

Allain and coworkers [1] reported the results of fifty-eight shoulders that underwent the Latarjet operation followed for an average of 143 months. None of the patients had recurrent dislocation, six patients had apprehension with regard to possible dislocation, and one had occasional subluxation. They found that the best results were in the group of patients in which the lateral edge graft was placed flush with the articular surface of the glenoid. If it was placed medial to this position there was an increased risk of dislocation or subluxation, and if it was placed lateral there was an increased risk of dislocation arthropathy.

While the results of coracoid transfer procedures for chronic anterior shoulder instability are known in terms of recurrence, the results in terms of apprehension have been rarely reported. Collin et al. [11] reported prospectively the results of a consecutive series of 74 patients treated with the Latarjet technique for anterior shoulder instability after an average follow-up of 50 months. Although the subjective satisfaction rate was 85 % and the failure rate 9 % (dislocation or subluxation), they found an unusually high rate of persistent apprehension. The apprehension correlated with early recovery of external rotation. For this reason they recommend adding Neer capsuloplasty to Latarjet coracoid block in patients with hyperlaxity associated with chronic anterior shoulder instability.

There are not head-to-head prospective studies comparing the results of coracoid transfer techniques versus Bankart repair in the literature. However, Hovelius et al. [18] reported recently a study at long-term follow-up of a retrospective analysis of 88 consecutive shoulders treated with a Bankart repair that were compared with a cohort of 97 shoulders managed with the Bristow procedure and followed prospectively. Results were significantly better after the Bristow than after Bankart repair with respect to postoperative stability and subjective evaluation. The external rotation lag was inferior in the group of patients managed with the Bankart operation.

The reports on the results of arthroscopic coracoid transfer procedures are still very scant and have a short- or mid-term follow-up. Lafosse and Boyle [26] reported prospectively their results of the first 100 shoulders undergoing all-arthroscopic Latarjet shoulder stabilization. At a mean follow-up of 26 months patient reported outcomes revealed 91 % excellent scores and 9 % good, with quick return to work and sports, satisfactory graft position in 78 % of the cases, and low complication rate. Boileau and co-workers reported in 2010 [5] the early the results of the arthroscopic Bankart-Bristow-Latarjet procedure. After a mean follow-up of 16 months, there were neither recurrences nor neurological complications, but conversion to open surgery was needed in 6 patients (12 %). Both groups warn on the technical difficulty of the procedure, and recommend restricting its use to those surgeons with good anatomic knowledge, and advanced arthroscopic skills. The senior author has recently reported the learning curve of the all-arthroscopic Latarjet technique, and found that the surgical time decreases significantly after the first 10 cases and that subscapularis split and coroacoid passage and fixation into the glenohumeral joint were the most difficult steps of the procedure. The position of the graft was excellent or good in 96 % of the cases as assessed with computed tomography [9].

There are several reports in the literature evaluating the results of the Latarjet procedure in specific populations with characteristics that make them not amenable of Bankart repair due to their higher failure rate. Burkhart et al. showed the efficacy of the congruent-arc Latarjet reconstruction in 47 patients with antero-inferior instability and significant glenoid bone loss or engaging Hill-Sachs lesion [7]. They had only a 4.9 % (four dislocations and 1 subluxation) recurrence rate at a mean follow-up of 59 months, and conclude that Latarjet is the procedure of choice in this group of patients. The group Lyonnais also achieved excellent results with the Latarjet in patients participating in collision sports, and reported excellent results with quick return to sporting activity in a series of soccer and rugby players [10, 30], although the rate of apprehension in this last group was 14 %. They also reported satisfactory outcomes in selected cases of anterior shoulder instability associated to full-thickness rotator cuff tears. The results improved in those patients in whom the cuff tear could be repaired [22]. However, the same group reported unacceptable rates of re-dislocation after surgery in patients with poorly controlled epilepsy [33]. All theses patients were diagnosed of anterior shoulder instability and had large bone defects at the glenoid and humeral head. Postoperative re-dislocations occurred during seizures, and the authors strongly recommend controlling epilepsy prior to stabilization surgery planning.

Concerning revision stabilization surgery, Schmid and associates [34] obtained a 2 % dislocation rate in a series of 49 consecutive patients undergoing Latarjet operation for recurrence of anterior shoulder instability after operative repair. No shoulder redislocated, subluxations recurred in two patients, and five patients reported slight, unspecified shoulder symptoms. Forty-three shoulders (88 %) were subjectively graded as excellent or good. The authors conclude that the Latarjet procedure is effective in postoperative shoulder stability.

4.4   Complications of Coracoid Transfer Techniques

The usual criticisms made to coracoid transfer techniques are that it constitutes a non-anatomic reconstruction of the shoulder with a risk of neurovascular injury, altering the subscapularis function or increasing the risk of developing a gleno-humeral osteoarthritis (dislocation arthropathy).

Shah et al. [36] recently reported a worrisome 25 % complication rate at short-term follow-up for the Latarjet procedure, including a 6 % infection rate, an 8 % instability recurrence rate, and a 10 % rate of neurologic injury. Some concerns have raised from the significant alterations found in certain anatomic studies in the relationships of the musculocutaneous and axillary nerves, which may make them vulnerable to injury during revision surgery or from the risk of damaging the supraescapular nerve with the screws used to fix the graft [14, 24]. European series, however, have not reported remarkable rates of neurovascular injuries, and the have been usually transient and resolved uneventfully when present, even those occurring during arthroscopic surgery [1, 9, 25, Boileau et al. 2012]. In fact, the complications reported by Shah et al. [36] occurred in a specific series of cases of revision surgery.

Isokinetic studies analysing the subscapularis function after coracoid transfer procedures have found that the muscular strength is recovered within the first 6–12 months of surgery, and shows no differences when compared to the pre-injury level [12, 31]. Our group evaluated the isokinetic performance and structural integrity of subscapularis after all arthroscopic Latarjet, and found no differences compared to a control group paired with regard to sex and age [13].

Dislocation arthropathy of the shoulder after surgical treatment of recurrent anterior dislocation with bone block procedures has been a subject of discussion. Allain et al. [1] first underlined the importance of the placement of the coracoid bone graft in the axial plane, and found a superior risk of dislocation arthropathy in those patients in whom the graft had been fixed lateral to the glenoid surface. Hovelius and co-workers [19] assessed radiographically the evolution of dislocation arthropathy at long-term follow-up in 118 shoulders operated with the Bristow technique for anterior instability. Dislocation arthropathy was found on ordinary anteroposterior views in 46 of 115 shoulders (mild in 39, moderate in 5, and severe in 2). The presence of arthropathy was related to the age of the patient. Global assessment of the operative result was not related to arthropathy at follow-up.

References

1. Allain J, Goutallier D, Glorion C (1998) Long-term results of the Latarjet procedure for the treatment of anterior instability of the shoulder. J Bone Joint Surg Am 80(6):841–852
2. Banas MP, Dalldorf PG, Sebastianelli WJ et al (1993) Long-term follow-up of the modified Bristow procedure. Am J Sports Med 21(5):666–671
3. Boileau P, Villalba M, Hery JY et al (2006) Risk factors for recurrence of shoulder instability after arthroscopic Bankart repair. J Bone Joint Surg Br 88:1755–1763
4. Boileau P, Bicknell RT, El Fegoun AB et al (2007) Arthroscopic Bristow procedure for anterior instability in shoulders with a stretched or deficient capsule: the "belt-and-suspenders" operative technique and preliminary results. Arthroscopy 23(6):593–601
5. Boileau P, Mercier N, Roussanne Y et al (2010) Arthroscopic Bankart-Bristow-Latarjet procedure: the development and early results of a safe and reproducible technique. Arthroscopy 26(11):1434–1450
6. Burkhart SS, De Beer JF (2000) Traumatic glenohumeral bone defects and their relationship to failure of arthroscopic Bankart repairs: significance of the inverted- pear glenoid and the humeral engaging Hill-Sachs lesion. Arthroscopy 16:677–694
7. Burkhart SS, De Beer JF, Barth JR et al (2007) Results of modified Latarjet reconstruction in patients with anteroinferior instability and significant bone loss. Arthroscopy 23:1033–1041
8. Calvo E, Granizo JJ, Fernández-Yruegas D (2005) Criteria for arthroscopic treatment of anterior instability of the shoulder. J Bone Joint Surg Br 87:677–683
9. Calvo E, Morcillo D, Foruria AM (2012) Arthroscopic Latarjet: the learning curve. In: Abstract book. 24th congress of the european society for surgery of the shoulder and elbow, Dubrovnik (Croatia), 19–22 September 2012
10. Cerciello S, Edwards TB, Walch G (2012) Chronic anterior glenohumeral instability in soccer players: results for a series of 28 shoulders treated with the Latarjet procedure. J Orthop Traumatol 13(4):197–202
11. Collin P, Rochcongar P, Thomazeau H (2007) Treatment of chronic anterior shoulder instability using a coracoid bone block (Latarjet procedure): 74 cases. Rev Chir Orthop Reparatrice Appar Mot 93(2):126–132
12. Edouard P, Beguin L, Degache F et al (2012) Recovery of rotators strength after Latarjet surgery. Int J Sports Med 33(9):749–755
13. Foruria AM, Morcillo D, Bermejo G et al (2012) Subscapularis structural integrity and function after arthroscopioc Latarjet: clinical, isokinetic and imaging study. In: Abstract book. 24th congress of the european society for surgery of the shoulder and elbow, Dubrovnik (Croatia), 19–22 September 2012
14. Freehill MT, Srikumaran U, Archer KR et al (2012) The Latarjet coracoid process transfer procedure: alterations in the neurovascular structures. J Shoulder Elbow Surg Sep 1 [Epub ahead of print]
15. Goudie EB, Murray IR, Robinson CM (2012) Instability of the shoulder following epilepsy. J Bone Joint Surg Br 94(6):721–728
16. Helfet AJ (1958) Coracoid transplantation for recurring dislocation of the shoulder. J Bone Joint Surg Br 40:198–202
17. Hovelius L, Körner L, Lundberg B et al (1983) The coracoid transfer for recurrent dislocation of the shoulder. Technical aspects of the Bristow-Latarjet procedure. J Bone Joint Surg Am 65(7):926–934
18. Hovelius LK, Sandström BC, Sundgren K et al (2004) One hundred eighteen Bristow-Latarjet repairs for recurrent anterior dislocation of the shoulder prospectively followed for fifteen years: study I—clinical results. J Shoulder Elbow Surg 13(5):509–516
19. Hovelius LK, Sandström BC, Saebo M (2006) One hundred eighteen Bristow-Latarjet repairs for recurrent anterior dislocation of the shoulder prospectively followed for fifteen years: study II-the evolution of dislocation arthropathy. J Shoulder Elbow Surg 15(3):279–289

20. Hovelius L, Vikerfors O, Olofsson A et al (2011) Bristow-Latarjet and Bankart: a comparative study of shoulder stabilization 185 shoulders during a seventeen-year follow-up. J Shoulder Elbow Surg 20(7):1095–1101
21. Hovelius LK, Sandström BC, Olofsson A (2012) The effect of capsular repair, bone block healing, and position on the results of the Bristow-Latarjet procedure (study III): long-term follow-up in 319 shoulders. J Shoulder Elbow Surg 21(5):647–660
22. Jouve F, Graveleau N, Nové-Josserand L et al (2008) Recurrent anterior instability of the shoulder associated with full thickness rotator cuff tear: results of surgical treatment. Rev Chir Orthop Reparatrice Appar Mot 94(7):659–669
23. Kim SH, Ha KI, Cho YB et al (2003) Arthroscopic anterior stabilization of the shoulder: two to six-year follow-up. J Bone Joint Surg 85:1511–1518
24. Lädermann A, Denard PJ, Burkhart SS (2012) Injury of the suprascapular nerve during latarjet procedure: an anatomic study. Arthroscopy 28(3):316–321
25. Lafosse L, Lejeune E, Bouchard A et al (2007) The arthroscopic Latarjet procedure for the treatment of anterior shoulder instability. Arthroscopy 23(11):1242, e1241–e1245
26. Lafosse L, Boyle S (2010) Arthroscopic Latarjet procedure. J Shoulder Elbow Surg 19:2–12
27. Latarjet M (1954) Treatment of recurrent dislocation of the shoulder. Lyon Chir 49:994–997
28. Mead NC, Sweeney HJ (1964) Bristow procedure (letter). Spectator July 9
29. Mohtadi NG, Bitar IJ, Sasyniuk TM et al (2005) Arthroscopic versus open repair for traumatic anterior shoulder instability: a meta-analysis. Arthroscopy 16:677–694
30. Neyton L, Young A, Dawidziak B et al (2012) Surgical treament of anterior instability in rugby union players: clinical and radiographic results of the Latarjet-Patte procedure with minimum 5-year follow-up. J Shoulder Elbow Surg 21(12):1721–1727
31. Paladini P, Merolla G, De Santis E et al (2012) Long-term subscapularis strength assessment after Bristow-Latarjet procedure: isometric study. J Shoulder Elbow Surg 21(1):42–47
32. Purchase RJ, Wolf EM, Hobgood ER et al (2008) Hill-Sachs "remplissage": an arthroscopic solution for the engaging Hill-Sachs lesion. Arthroscopy 24:723–726
33. Raiss P, Lin A, Mizuno N et al (2012) Results of the Latarjet procedure for recurrent anterior dislocation of the shoulder in patients with epilepsy. J Bone Joint Surg Br 94(9):1260–1264
34. Schmid SL, Farshad M, Catanzaro S, Gerber C (2012) The Latarjet procedure for the treatment of recurrence of anterior instability of the shoulder after operative repair: a retrospective case series of forty-nine consecutive patients. J Bone Joint Surg Am 94:e75(1–7)
35. Schroder DT, Provencher MT, Mologne TS et al (2006) The modified Bristow procedure for anterior shoulder instability: 26-year outcomes in Naval Academy midshipmen. Am J Sports Med 34(5):778–786
36. Shah AA, Butler RB, Romanowski J et al (2012) Short-term complications of the Latarjet procedure. J Bone Joint Surg Am 94(6):495–501
37. Thelu C, Ohl X, Elofi O, et al (2012). Arthroscopic Bristow-Latarjet procedure using suture endo-button technique. In: Abstract book. 24th congress of the european society for surgery of the shoulder and elbow, Dubrovnik (Croatia), 19–22 September 2012
38. Torg JS, Balduini FC, Bonci C et al (1987) A modified Bristow-Helfet-May procedure for recurrent dislocation and subluxation of the shoulder. Report of two hundred and twelve cases. J Bone Joint Surg Am 69(6):904–913
39. Wredmark T, Törnkvist H, Johansson C et al (1992) Long-term functional results of the modified Bristow procedure for recurrent dislocations of the shoulder. Am J Sports Med 20(2):157–161

Arthroscopic Coracoid Transfer

5

Michael T. Freehill, Sandeep Mannava, Austin Vo,
Daniel G. Schwartz and Laurent Lafosse

5.1 Introduction

The best operative procedure to address anterior recurrent instability in both the index and revision setting remains a subject of orthopaedic surgical debate. Though many published reports propose treatment algorithms to aid the surgeon in operative technique selection; ultimately, institutional precedent and surgeon experience often dictate the procedure performed. This report briefly describes the arthroscopic Latarjet procedure (ALP), presents indications for the procedure—including the trends of the senior author in utilizing the ALP technique in his high volume, shoulder only practice—and summarizes the state of the current shoulder instability literature, as well as future trends.

5.2 Operative Interventions to Address Shoulder Instability

When addressing anterior recurrent instability of the shoulder following a primary dislocation event, multiple treatment options have been described, including: non-operative management, open or arthroscopic stabilization, and bone block/transfer procedures. If one considers humeral head bony loss, even more options are

M. T. Freehill (✉) · S. Mannava
Department of Orthopaedic Surgery, Division of Sports Medicine, Wake Forest University School of Medicine, Medical Center Boulevard, Winston-Salem, NC 27157, USA
e-mail: freehill@wakehealth.edu

A. Vo · D. G. Schwartz · L. Lafosse
Alps Surgery Institute, Clinique Generale, Annecy, France

S. F. Brockmeier et al. (eds.), *Surgery of Shoulder Instability*,
DOI: 10.1007/978-3-642-38100-3_5, © ISAKOS 2013

available including; remplissage, humeral head allograft, disimpaction of the Hill-Sachs, humeral rotational osteotomy, prosthetic reconstruction, and Latarjet procedures [1–6]. The chief determinant for surgical procedure choice in operatively addressing anterior shoulder instability remains surgeon preference. Numerous factors including surgeon experience, surgical training, and patient characteristics such as: soft tissue quality, glenoid or humeral head bony status, previous surgical intervention, and activity level influence the operative procedure chosen to address recurrent anterior shoulder instability. Several published reports have proposed an algorithmic approach to deciding upon surgical intervention offered to the patient for shoulder instability [2, 7–9]. Surgical options in these algorithms include both arthroscopic and open repair, as well as bony transfer or augmentation procedures [2, 7–9].

In most instances, recurrent shoulder instability can be addressed surgically with either an arthroscopic or open Bankart repair, to address the most common lesion associated with a shoulder dislocation, a capsulolabral avulsion from the glenoid rim [10]. However, this approach to operatively addressing shoulder instability becomes problematic when performed on patients who have more extensive soft tissue injuries such as capsular attenuation, complex labral disruptions that render the labrum dysfunctional, or humeral avulsion of glenohumeral ligament (HAGL) lesions. In these cases of extensive soft tissue injury following shoulder dislocation, operative repair of the labrum to the glenoid rim often fails to adequately restore shoulder stability.

Similarly, inferior clinical results have been associated with a capsulolabral repair, when used in cases with the concomitant glenoid bony deficiency [6, 11]. Historically, Latarjet procedures have been reserved for shoulder instability cases in which the patient has greater than 25–30 % of glenoid bone loss. This critical loss of bone has been demonstrated to lead to a loss of glenohumeral articular conformity, or glenoid tracking; thereby causing instability [12–14].

Recent reports in the literature have suggested an expanded indication, beyond critical amounts of glenoid bone loss, for performing a Latarjet procedure in cases of recurrent shoulder instability. In particular, younger patients (<20 years) and those involved in overhead or contact sports were followed for several years and determined to have inadequate operative treatment when only capsulolabral repairs were performed. Balg and Boileau [9] described a 10-point pre-operative instability severity index score (ISIS) and determined a score greater than 6 points had an unacceptable recurrent instability risk of 70 % when only capsulolabral repairs were performed. They concluded an arthroscopic Bankart repair is contraindicated in these cases; instead the study suggests that a Bristow-Latarjet procedure may be more appropriate in addressing the recurrent instability [9]. Similarly, Young et al. reported successful use of the Latarjet procedure when operating upon patients with recurrent anterior instability, with or without hyperlaxity, and with or without glenoid and/or humeral bone loss [15].

5.3   Brief Description of the Arthroscopic Latarjet Procedure (ALP)

Lafosse et al. has previously described an arthroscopic Latarjet procedure (ALP) [16, 17]. This technique affords the benefits of a bone block procedure in a less invasive manner than the open procedure. Additionally, the procedure offers the potential for reduced scar tissue, improved cosmesis, decreased post-op pain, and greater subjective patient satisfaction [16, 17]. The ALP procedure technique will be briefly presented in this report; for a more complete description of the procedure the reader is referred to the original manuscript by Lafosse et al. [16, 17].

To perform the arthroscopic Latarjet, the patient is positioned in the beach chair position. Superficial surgical landmarks and portal placement used to perform ALP are depicted in Fig. 5.1. After a focused diagnostic shoulder arthroscopic evaluation is performed, attention is turned to antero-inferior glenoid preparation with removal of the labrum and capsulectomy in preparation for graft placement. Following initial glenoid preparation, the rotator interval is opened to gain access to the coracoid and conjoint tendon. The coracoacromial ligament is detached, while care is taken not to disrupt the conjoint tendon. The rotator interval is further opened through an additional anterolateral portal (E), this same portal is used to complete the coracoid preparation, as well as for exposure of the anterior and posterior subscapularis. Additional infero-lateral (J), inferior (I), and medial (M) portals are then created to aid in the coracoid process harvest. During the coracoid harvest, the pectoralis minor is resected from the coracoid; while performing this step, the brachial plexus, as well as the musculocutaneous nerve are at risk. After complete coracoid exposure, an

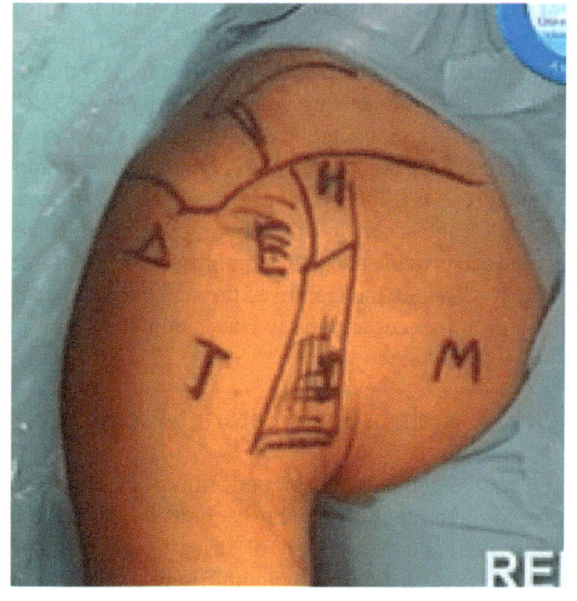

Fig. 5.1 Surgical landmarks and portal sites used for arthroscopic coracoid transfer sugery. Reproduced with permission from L. Laffosse, MD ©

additional portal (H) is created above the coracoid in order to gain access for pre-drilling the coracoid osteotomy. A commercial available drill guide has been developed to aide in the coracoid harvest process. Care should be taken during this portion of the procedure, as the cephalic vein is at risk during the introduction of the drill guide. The process of coracoid preparation requires creating multiple drill holes over a K-wire guide that are additionally tapped. Over the K-wire guides, a 'top-hat' washer is placed into the coracoid and then a burr is used to create a ring stress riser to help protect propagation of the osteotomy towards the proximal hole in the coracoid. After the ring is completed, the osteotomy can be completed with a chisel through the H-portal.

Attention is then turned toward creating a subscapularis split, between the middle third and inferior third of the tendon. After verification of correct split location through various portals, a split in the subscapularis is created using electrocautery. The coracoid transfer is then undertaken, where the coracoid is retrieved and fixed to a cannula by two screws that are placed through the top hats into bone. The coracoid is then fully mobilized with the remainder of soft tissue attachments being released. Prior to placement of the coracoid to the glenoid, gentle burring of the surfaces that will be opposed is performed on both the glenoid and on the coracoid graft. To facilitate the mobilization of the coracoid graft towards the glenoid, the arm is placed in internal rotation and forward flexion, thereby releasing the conjoint tendon and opening the subscapularis split. The cannula is used to joy-stick the coracoid graft into proper position on the glenoid, a process facilitated by a switching stick through another posterior portal to aid in retraction of the soft tissues.

The final step of the ALP is coracoid fixation. Prior to attempting coracoid fixation, the scapula is retracted posteriorly by placement of a Healix 6, 5 tap screw in the site of the coracoid osteotomy, which is later used as a joy-stick. The graft is then positioned and two K-wires are used to drill through the graft, glenoid, and finally through the posterior shoulder skin. These K-wires firmly provisionally affix the graft, the cannulated screw is then removed and a hole is drilled with a 3.2 mm cannulated drill, starting with the inferior hole. The screw length is measured is the standard fashion using the drill bit just as the posterior glenoid is perforated (in our experience this measurement is typically 34–36 mm and we utilize partially cannulated screws). The inferior screw is then inserted and the process is repeated once again for the superior screw (Fig. 5.2). Care must be taken to alternately tighten the screws to provide adequate compression without fracturing or medializing the graft. The K-wires are then removed through the cannula, the graft position is checked, and any prominences are gently corrected with a burr.

5.4   Arthroscopic Latarjet Procedure Indications

Operative indications for performing an arthroscopic Latarjet procedure (ALP) based upon the senior author's clinical experience include recurrent anterior instability, defined as a history of at least one dislocation event followed by recurrent episodes of instability including: repeat dislocation, subluxation, or a subjective

Fig. 5.2 The coracoid bone graft being placed arthroscopically at the anteroinferior glenoid rim. Reproduced with permission from L. Laffosse, MD ©

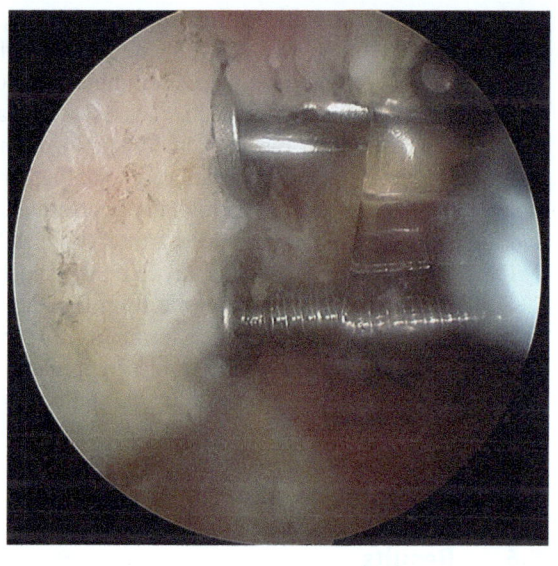

sensation of apprehension. Additionally, the presence of any glenoid bone involvement (fracture or eburnation), an engaging Hill-Sachs lesion demonstrated dynamically at the time of arthroscopy, a combination of glenoid and humeral bone loss [18], a failed previous stabilization procedure, or the presence of a humeral avulsion of the glenohumeral ligament (HAGL lesion) are all indications for an ALP. Finally, if at the time of an attempted primary arthroscopic Bankart repair, it is noted the soft tissue integrity is poor, conversion to an ALP is performed.

Of note, the senior author still performs arthroscopic Bankart stabilization in cases of anterior instability when the symptoms are minor and limited to apprehension or subluxation without complete dislocation. Frequently, this type of minor or limited instability is dependent upon the integrity of the inferior glenohumeral ligament (IGHL) and the labrum. If the labrum is not torn, the ring keeps its elastic concentric forces after healing around the glenoid, like a tie around a wheel. At our institution, this type of lesion is reparable with the potential for good functional results.

5.5 Senior Author Experience

The surgical logs of the senior author (L.L.) were retrospectively reviewed from January 2003 through December of 2012. All arthroscopic Latarjet procedures (ALP) performed during this period of time were analyzed. All procedures were performed at Alps Surgery Institute, Clinique Generale (Annecy, France) (n = 355) or Clinique Generale-Beaulieu (Geneva, Switzerland) (n = 30). The ALP technique has been previously described and published by the senior author [16, 17] and he continues making minor technical modifications to the procedure, to improve efficiency based on his extensive experience performing the operation.

At the time of the initial arthroscopic evaluation, prior to the start of the ALP procedure, if the injury was determined to be an isolated labral avulsion from the glenoid rim in a primary setting, with minimal concomitant pathology, a standard Bankart procedure was performed. All cases were analyzed to determine if an open or arthroscopic Bankart repair shoulder stabilization surgery was previously performed. Previous open versus arthroscopic Bankart repair groups were further analyzed to determine if the senior author performed the failed initial stabilization, and the amount of time from index arthroscopic stabilization to ALP.

Patients were excluded from analysis if they underwent additional procedures to their affected unstable shoulder aside from Bankart surgery. Thus, failed Bankart repairs are the only prior shoulder instability surgery performed prior to revision ALP surgery. One patient in 2009 had two previous open Bankart repairs and one patient in 2010 had 4 arthroscopic Bankart failures, neither were performed by the senior author. These patients were analyzed as though they had failed Bankart surgery once. Data were analyzed using descriptive statistics.

5.6   Results

Over the 9 year period, 385 arthroscopic Latarjet procedures were performed by the senior author. In the setting of an ALP for a failed Bankart repair, the mean age of patients undergoing an ALP was 28.40 years (range 15–63) with 13 females (20.6 %) and 50 males (79.4 %). Fifty-one were right hand dominant (81 %) and 12 were left hand dominant (19 %). The dominant arm was the affected unstable side 51.0 % (28/55) of the time. The operative side was the contralateral side left in 27 (42.9 %) and right in 36 (57.1 %).

There was a steady annual increase in the number of arthroscopic Latarjet surgeries performed by the senior author (Fig. 5.3). The number rose from one procedure being performed in 2003 to 78 being performed in 2011. Sixty-nine ALPs were performed in the setting of a failed previous Bankart repair, representing 17.92 % of the total ALPs performed during the study period (Fig. 5.4). In the senior author's practice, most ALPs were performed for primary operative management of shoulder instability (range of 1–63 primary ALP performed

Fig. 5.3 Number of arthroscopic Latarjet procedures (ALP) performed annually by the senior author

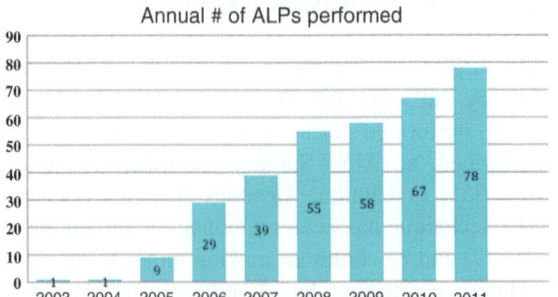

Fig. 5.4 Number of arthroscopic Latarjet procedures (ALP) performed annually for primary instability repair and previous Bankart revisions

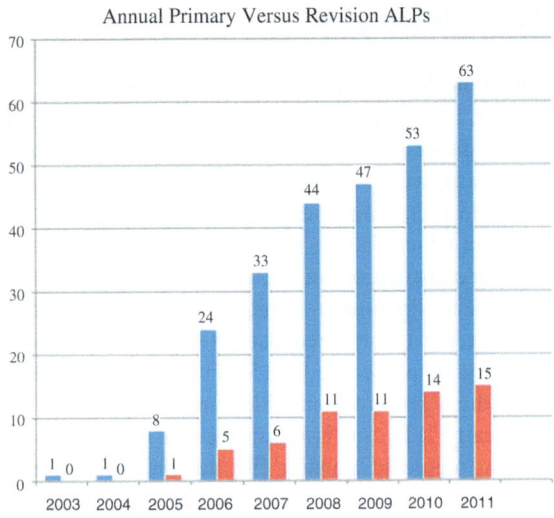

Annual Primary Versus Revision ALPs

between 2003 and 2012, Fig. 5.4). The mean percentage of ALPs being performed for a failed Bankart annually ranged from 11 to 21 % annually, with the number of failed open versus arthroscopic Bankart repairs being 8 (12.70 %) and 55 (87.30 %) respectively (Fig. 5.5). The senior author personally performed 29 of 55 (52.73 %) of the failed arthroscopic Bankart repairs and the mean time to revision surgery was 50 months (range 3–168 months) in this cohort of patients.

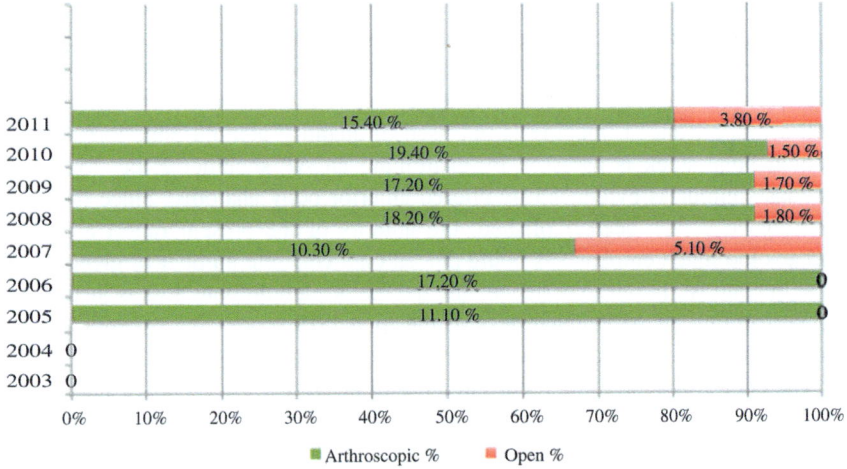

Fig. 5.5 Percentage of failed open versus arthroscopic Bankart repairs undergoing an ALP per year

5.7   Discussion

There has been an annual increase in the number of ALPs performed by the senior author. Interestingly, this increasing trend demonstrates performing an ALP as the index procedure for the treatment of recurrent anterior shoulder instability (Fig. 5.4), which contrasts published shoulder instability treatment algorithms [2, 7–9]. In fact, many published reports advocate reserving bony reconstruction to cases in which there is glenoid bone loss of 20 to 30 % [12–14, 19–24]. However, bony reconstruction for shoulder instability aside from instances of bone defect has precedent. Previous reports, mainly from France, describe different indices for considering Latarjet reconstruction of the glenoid, with expanded indications for the surgical procedure [9, 15]. The senior author advocates for bony reconstruction to address recurrent shoulder instability, as he performs ALPs for an ISIS of 2 (typically ISIS > 6 is considered at high risk of recurrent dislocation thus warranting coracoid transfer [9]. Justification for this approach is based upon the observation that the structural integrity of the glenohumeral ligaments is often altered after dislocation events, which may not always be apparent macroscopically. Thus, capsulolabral repair alone may not provide sufficient reconstruction for the difficult to observe extensive pathology that underlies the patient's shoulder instability.

Of the 55 revision ALPs performed between 2003 and 2011, the senior author was responsible for performing 29 (52.7 %) of the failed index Bankart procedures. The senior author's preferred technique employed for Bankart repair is the Cassiopeia technique, which is regarded as a strong and durable arthroscopic repair [25, 26]. In this cohort of patients, the time to revision surgery was 50 months, with a large range of 3–168 months. Long-term follow-up studies are required to specifically address the integrity and durability of Bankart repair surgery for addressing shoulder instability; however, the data from the present report suggest variability in patient outcomes after Bankart repair.

The original published recommendation of ISIS > 6 was the threshold required to perform a coracoid transfer [9]. When critically examining the limitations of the ISIS score, advanced imaging is not used to quantify glenoid bone loss. Instead, glenoid bone stock is assessed by examining an AP shoulder X-ray for loss of osseous contour as evidenced by altered anterior bony anatomy. Since the report by Balg et al. has been published, the authors of the present report argue that perhaps too much emphasis is being placed on a concrete number of glenoid bone loss. In contrast, in our experience, any degree of glenoid bone loss is justification for performing an ALP, regardless of the total ISIS score. The exception to this indication is the occasional acute case of anterior shoulder instability.

The choice of addressing recurrent anterior instability after a failed stabilization attempt is based on the structural cause of the failure. Risk factors implicated in failure of the index shoulder stabilization procedure include: insufficient number of suture anchors used, improper placement of the suture anchors, younger patient age, ligamentous laxity, capsular stretching, participation in contact sports, and bony loss of the glenoid or humerus [6, 9, 12, 13, 27–31]. Meehan and Petersen reported that a surgical history of two or more failed shoulder instability procedures and bony Bankart lesions confer higher risk of ultimately requiring an open shoulder stabilization procedure [32].

In the literature, open stabilization techniques remain the gold standard for shoulder stabilization surgery, with reported recurrent dislocation rates ranging from 0 to 7 % [31, 33–37]. However the open surgical techniques are known to restrict shoulder motion, particularly external rotation [34–38]. Despite existing data on open repair, arthroscopic shoulder stabilization surgical techniques are gaining popularity. Recurrent dislocation rates after arthroscopic stabilization appear to be on the decline with recent reported dislocation rates ranging from 4 to 19 %. This decline is likely a result of improved arthroscopic surgical technique and advances in arthroscopic technology [11, 30, 31, 33, 39–42]. Owens et al. reported the total number of Bankart procedures performed from 2003 to 2008 entered into the American Board of Orthopaedic Surgery database by surgical candidates for oral certification [43]. From 2003 to 2005, 71.2 % of Bankart repairs were performed arthroscopically, this number increased to 87.7 % from 2006 to 2008, and once again increased to 90 % in 2008. Furthermore, in 2008, both fellowship trained and non-fellowship trained sports medicine surgeons were performing 90 % arthroscopic Bankart repairs. These data may reflect the rising popularity of arthroscopic Bankart repair, as well as a possible decreased comfort of recent U.S. residency trained orthopaedic surgery graduates in performing open stabilization procedures [43].

Examining our data, the number of ALPs increased annually (Fig. 5.3); however, the percentage of revision ALPs performed for failed Bankart repair remained relatively constant between 11 and 21 % in 2005–2011 (Fig. 5.5). The data reflect that arthroscopic Bankart repairs are more likely to be revised by ALPs than open Bankart repairs (Fig. 5.5); however, this observation may be due to the arthroscopic Bankart technique being more popular and commonly performed when compared to open surgery [43].

Redfern and Burks reported a survey of the attendees of the 2009 Metcalf Memorial Arthroscopy Association of North America course and noted 71 % of respondents performed arthroscopic Bankart repair "almost always" for shoulder instability and 59 % had never performed a bone-graft procedure for anterior shoulder instability [44]. With a reported recurrent shoulder instability rate as high as 67 % after arthroscopic stabilization in patients with glenoid bone loss, there may be an increased need for revision shoulder instability surgery in the near future [6, 11].

Critics of the Latarjet procedure claim a distortion of the natural shoulder anatomy, as the coracoid process is transferred to the glenoid. Additionally, the pectoralis minor, as well as the coracoacromial ligament, is released. Shortcomings and complications of the Latarjet procedure include: the procedure not addressing capsular laxity; nonunion of the transferred coracoid; hardware (screw) complications; post-operative glenohumeral arthrosis; loss of shoulder range of motion; weakening of the subscapularis; and increased difficulty when attempting to revise a failed Latarjet operation [45–48]. When performing a Latarjet procedure, a muscle splitting approach has been associated with decreased post-operative subscapularis dysfunction [49–51]. Young et al. did not report a loss in external rotation after their patients underwent the Latarjet procedure[15].

Young et al. additionally reported the results for 2000 Latarjet procedures with instability recurrence rates less than 1 %, while 98 % of patients in their series reported their surgical result as excellent or good [15]. Others have reported similar favorable results after Latarjet shoulder stability surgery [48, 52–55].

The minimally invasive ALP has several advantages when compared to a traditional open Latarjet procedure including the ability for the patient to have immediate postoperative range of motion rehabilitation, including external rotation. Early post-operative rehabilitation is postulated to improve post-surgical motion in patients who have undergone the ALP. Lafosse et al. reported that 35 patients from the first 100 ALPs performed demonstrated an average loss of 18 degrees of external rotation compared with the opposite shoulder [17]. Since those initial surgeries were performed, modifications have been made to the ALP technique and the senior author believes ALP patients undergo minimal losses in motion after surgery; however, long-term studies are needed to confirm this post-operative observation. In the first 100 ALPs performed by the senior author, 80 % of the patients describe their result as excellent, 8 % as good, and 2 % disappointed at an 18 month follow-up. In this same series, the authors notes that the learning curve for performing ALP is substantial [17].

The shoulder joint capsule is not repaired or augmented during an ALP, which differs from the open Latarjet technique; but the critical nature of capsular repair remains unknown. Additionally, when performing an ALP, the coracoacromial ligament is not repaired to the capsule, yet long-term consequences of not performing this repair also remains unknown. Despite these differences in surgical technique between the open and arthroscopic Latarjet surgery, the principles of restoring stability via the triple blocking effect are postulated to apply to the ALP.

The material presented in this manuscript, as well as the interpretation of the literature must be considered in the proper context. The senior author has a highly specialized, large volume shoulder surgery practice, with particular expertise in complex arthroscopic shoulder surgery. The purpose of this article is not to persuade the reader to perform the arthroscopic Latarjet procedure or support its utilization versus other procedure choices. This manuscript represents observations from one surgeon's high volume practice, which may stimulate debate as to how surgical repair of recurrent shoulder instability may be performed. Undoubtedly, in the United States, performing an ALP for an index procedure in the absence of osseous involvement would be considered by many as 'too aggressive', as there is limited literature supporting utilization of this technique routinely. The long-term results of the ALP will require continued monitoring and reporting prior to widespread adoption of this surgical technique.

5.8   Conclusion

The ALP offers a surgical option for recurrent anterior instability. Despite the annual increase in the number of ALPs performed annually by the senior author, the percentage of failed Bankart repairs (presenting with a recurrent dislocation) addressed with an ALP procedure remained relatively constant throughout the study period. Since arthroscopic Bankart repairs have become an increasingly popular option for shoulder stability surgery and the data presented in this study suggest that arthroscopic Bankart repairs have a higher revision rate, the need for ALP procedures may increase in the future. Despite demonstrated success of the ALP procedure when performed by the senior author, it is recommended the procedure be performed by surgeons with sound anatomic knowledge, advanced arthroscopic skills, and familiarity with the specialized instrumentation.

References:

1. Yamamoto N et al (2009) Effect of an anterior glenoid defect on anterior shoulder stability: a cadaveric study. Am J Sports Med 37(5):949–954
2. Chen AL et al (2005) Management of bone loss associated with recurrent anterior glenohumeral instability. Am J Sports Med 33(6):912–925
3. Sekiya JK et al (2009) Hill-Sachs defects and repair using osteoarticular allograft transplantation: biomechanical analysis using a joint compression model. Am J Sports Med 37(12):2459–2466
4. Kaar SG et al (2010) Effect of humeral head defect size on glenohumeral stability: a cadaveric study of simulated Hill-Sachs defects. Am J Sports Med 38(3):594–599
5. Purchase RJ et al (2008) Hill-sachs "remplissage": an arthroscopic solution for the engaging hill-sachs lesion. Arthroscopy 24(6):723–726
6. Burkhart SS, De Beer JF (2000) Traumatic glenohumeral bone defects and their relationship to failure of arthroscopic Bankart repairs: significance of the inverted-pear glenoid and the humeral engaging Hill-Sachs lesion. Arthroscopy 16(7):677–694
7. Piasecki DP et al (2009) Glenoid bone deficiency in recurrent anterior shoulder instability: diagnosis and management. J Am Acad Orthop Surg 17(8):482–493
8. Mauro CS et al (2011) Failed anterior shoulder stabilization. J Shoulder Elbow Surg 20(8):1340–1350
9. Balg F, Boileau P (2007) The instability severity index score. A simple pre-operative score to select patients for arthroscopic or open shoulder stabilisation. J Bone Joint Surg Br 89(11):1470–1477
10. Hintermann B, Gachter A (1995) Arthroscopic findings after shoulder dislocation. Am J Sports Med 23(5):545–551
11. Boileau P et al (2006) Risk factors for recurrence of shoulder instability after arthroscopic Bankart repair. J Bone Joint Surg Am 88(8):1755–1763
12. Burkhart SS, Danaceau SM (2000) Articular arc length mismatch as a cause of failed bankart repair. Arthroscopy 16(7):740–744
13. Itoi E et al (2000) The effect of a glenoid defect on anteroinferior stability of the shoulder after Bankart repair: a cadaveric study. J Bone Joint Surg Am 82(1):35–46
14. Yamamoto N et al (2009) Effect of an anterior glenoid defect on anterior shoulder stability: a cadaveric study. Am J Sports Med 37(5):949–954
15. Young AA et al (2011) Open Latarjet procedure for management of bone loss in anterior instability of the glenohumeral joint. J Shoulder Elbow Surg 20(2 Suppl):S61–S69

16. Lafosse L et al (2007) The arthroscopic Latarjet procedure for the treatment of anterior shoulder instability. Arthroscopy 23(11):1242 e1-5
17. Lafosse L et al (2010) Arthroscopic latarjet procedure. Orthop Clin North Am 41(3):393–405
18. Yamamoto N et al (2007) Contact between the glenoid and the humeral head in abduction, external rotation, and horizontal extension: a new concept of glenoid track. J Shoulder Elbow Surg 16(5):649–656
19. Chuang TY, Adams CR, Burkhart SS (2008) Use of preoperative three-dimensional computed tomography to quantify glenoid bone loss in shoulder instability. Arthroscopy 24(4):376–382
20. Gerber C, Nyffeler RW (2002) Classification of glenohumeral joint instability. Clin Orthop Relat Res 400:65–76
21. Huijsmans PE et al (2007) Quantification of a glenoid defect with three-dimensional computed tomography and magnetic resonance imaging: a cadaveric study. J Shoulder Elbow Surg 16(6):803–899
22. Lo IK, Parten PM, Burkhart SS (2004) The inverted pear glenoid: an indicator of significant glenoid bone loss. Arthroscopy 20(2):169–174
23. Sugaya H et al (2003) Glenoid rim morphology in recurrent anterior glenohumeral instability. J Bone Joint Surg Am 85-A(5):878–884
24. Warner JJ et al (2006) Anatomical glenoid reconstruction for recurrent anterior glenohumeral instability with glenoid deficiency using an autogenous tricortical iliac crest bone graft. Am J Sports Med 34(2):205–212
25. Ahmad CS et al (2009) Evaluation of glenoid capsulolabral complex insertional anatomy and restoration with single- and double-row capsulolabral repairs. J Shoulder Elbow Surg 18(6):948–954
26. Lafosse L, Baier GP, Jost B (2006) Footprint fixation for arthroscopic reconstruction in anterior shoulder instability: the Cassiopeia double-row technique. Arthroscopy 22(2):231 e1-231 e6
27. Rowe CR, Zarins B, Ciullo JV (1984) Recurrent anterior dislocation of the shoulder after surgical repair. Apparent causes of failure and treatment. J Bone Joint Surg Am 66(2):159–168
28. Imhoff AB et al (2010) Arthroscopic repair of anterior-inferior glenohumeral instability using a portal at the 5:30-o'clock position: analysis of the effects of age, fixation method, and concomitant shoulder injury on surgical outcomes. Am J Sports Med 38(9):1795–1803
29. Bigliani LU et al (1998) Glenoid rim lesions associated with recurrent anterior dislocation of the shoulder. Am J Sports Med 26(1):41–55
30. Voos JE et al (2010) Prospective evaluation of arthroscopic Bankart repairs for anterior instability. Am J Sports Med 38(2):302–307
31. Bottoni CR et al (2006) Arthroscopic versus open shoulder stabilization for recurrent anterior instability: a prospective randomized clinical trial. Am J Sports Med 34(11):1730–1737
32. Meehan RE, Petersen SA (2005) Results and factors affecting outcome of revision surgery for shoulder instability. J Shoulder Elbow Surg 14(1):31–37
33. Fabbriciani C et al (2004) Arthroscopic versus open treatment of Bankart lesion of the shoulder: a prospective randomized study. Arthroscopy 20(5):456–462
34. Cole BJ et al (2000) Comparison of arthroscopic and open anterior shoulder stabilization. A two to six-year follow-up study. J Bone Joint Surg Am 82-A(8):1108–1114
35. Cole BJ, Warner JJ (2000) Arthroscopic versus open Bankart repair for traumatic anterior shoulder instability. Clin Sports Med 19(1):19–48
36. Kartus J et al (1998) Arthroscopic and open shoulder stabilization using absorbable implants. A clinical and radiographic comparison of two methods. Knee Surg Sports Traumatol Arthrosc 6(3):181–188
37. Rosenberg BN, Richmond JC, Levine WN (1995) Long-term followup of Bankart reconstruction. Incidence of late degenerative glenohumeral arthrosis. Am J Sports Med 23(5):538–544

38. Sperber A et al (2001) Comparison of an arthroscopic and an open procedure for posttraumatic instability of the shoulder: a prospective, randomized multicenter study. J Shoulder Elbow Surg 10(2):105–108
39. Kim SH et al (2003) Arthroscopic anterior stabilization of the shoulder: two to six-year follow-up. J Bone Joint Surg Am 85-A(8):1511–1518
40. Carreira DS et al (2006) A prospective outcome evaluation of arthroscopic Bankart repairs: minimum 2-year follow-up. Am J Sports Med 34(5):771–777
41. Flinkkila T et al (2010) Arthroscopic Bankart repair: results and risk factors of recurrence of instability. Knee Surg Sports Traumatol Arthrosc 18(12):1752–1758
42. Calvo E, Granizo JJ, Fernandez-Yruegas D (2005) Criteria for arthroscopic treatment of anterior instability of the shoulder: a prospective study. J Bone Joint Surg Br 87(5):677–683
43. Owens BD et al (2011) Surgical trends in Bankart repair: an analysis of data from the American Board of Orthopaedic Surgery certification examination. Am J Sports Med 39(9):1865–1869
44. Redfern J, Burks R (2009) 2009 survey results: surgeon practice patterns regarding arthroscopic surgery. Arthroscopy 25(12):1447–1452
45. Young DC, Rockwood CA Jr (1991) Complications of a failed Bristow procedure and their management. J Bone Joint Surg Am 73(7):969–981
46. Zuckerman JD, Matsen FA 3rd (1984) Complications about the glenohumeral joint related to the use of screws and staples. J Bone Joint Surg Am 66(2):175–180
47. Scheibel M et al (2004) Open reconstruction of anterior glenoid rim fractures. Knee Surg Sports Traumatol Arthrosc 12(6):568–573
48. Allain J, Goutallier D, Glorion C (1998) Long-term results of the Latarjet procedure for the treatment of anterior instability of the shoulder. J Bone Joint Surg Am 80(6):841–852
49. Maynou C, Cassagnaud X, Mestdagh H (2005) Function of subscapularis after surgical treatment for recurrent instability of the shoulder using a bone-block procedure. J Bone Joint Surg Br 87(8):1096–1101
50. Elkousy H et al (2010) Subscapularis function following the Latarjet coracoid transfer for recurrent anterior shoulder instability. Orthopedics 33(11):802
51. Paladini P et al (2012) Long-term subscapularis strength assessment after Bristow-Latarjet procedure: isometric study. J Shoulder Elbow Surg 21(1):42–47
52. Hovelius L et al (2004) One hundred eighteen Bristow-Latarjet repairs for recurrent anterior dislocation of the shoulder prospectively followed for fifteen years: study I–clinical results. J Shoulder Elbow Surg 13(5):509–516
53. Hovelius LK et al (2001) Long-term results with the Bankart and Bristow-Latarjet procedures: recurrent shoulder instability and arthropathy. J Shoulder Elbow Surg 10(5):445–452
54. Spoor AB, de Waal Malefijt J (2005) Long-term results and arthropathy following the modified Bristow-Latarjet procedure. Int Orthop 29(5):265–267
55. Collin P, Rochcongar P, Thomazeau H (2007) Treatment of chronic anterior shoulder instability using a coracoid bone block (Latarjet procedure): 74 cases. Rev Chir Orthop Reparatrice Appar Mot 93(2):126–132

Osteochondral Allograft Augmentation of the Glenoid for Instability with Bone Deficiency

6

Rachel M. Frank, John McNeil, Michael Hellman, Anthony A. Romeo and CDR Matthew T. Provencher

6.1   Introduction

Glenohumeral joint stability depends on both static and dynamic stabilizing factors. Static stabilizers include the osseous anatomy of the glenohumeral joint as well as the capsulolabral complex. Dynamic stabilizers include the rotator cuff (supraspinatous, infraspinatous, teres minor, and subscapularis) musculature as well as the long head of the biceps tendon (LHBT). A complex interaction between these factors is necessary for maintaining consistent centering of the humeral head onto the glenoid. The pathology most encountered in anterior shoulder instability is an avulsion of the anteroinferior glenoid labrum at its attachment to the inferior glenohumeral ligament (IGHL) complex, known as a Bankart lesion [1–4]. This lesion often occurs with avulsion of the capsular tissue from the glenoid rim. In

R. M. Frank · J. McNeil · M. Hellman · A. A. Romeo
Section of Shoulder and Elbow Surgery, Department of Orthopaedic Surgery,
Rush University Medical Center, 1611 West Harrison Street, Suite 300, Chicago,
IL 60612, USA
e-mail: Rmfrank3@gmail.com

J. McNeil
e-mail: jmcneil@ucsd.edu

M. Hellman
e-mail: mdhellman@gmail.com

A. A. Romeo
e-mail: shoulderelbowdoc@gmail.com

CDR M. T. Provencher (✉)
Surgery and Orthopaedics, USUHS, Orthopaedic Shoulder, Knee and Sports Surgery,
Department of Orthopaedic Surgery, Naval Medical Center San Diego, 34800 Bob Wilson
Dr. Ste 112, San Diego, CA 92134, USA
e-mail: matthew.provencher@med.navy.mil

S. F. Brockmeier et al. (eds.), *Surgery of Shoulder Instability*,
DOI: 10.1007/978-3-642-38100-3_6, © ISAKOS 2013

many cases, this injury occurs with fracture of the anteroinferior glenoid bone itself, known as a bony Bankart lesion. Historically, the goal of surgical intervention has been to restore a functional anteroinferior capsulolabral complex, however recent literature has proven the importance of addressing glenoid bone defects in an effort to prevent, or in many cases, treat, recurrent anteroinferior glenohumeral instability. Restoring glenoid congruency in cases of recurrent shoulder instability can be challenging as several factors including lesion size, location, and patient activity level, can influence which surgical procedure is most appropriate. A substantial amount of recent literature has been devoted to this topic, yet the treatment options still remain controversial. This manuscript will provide a review of the bone graft options currently available for restoring bony deficiency of the anteroinferior glenoid.

6.2   Epidemiology

The literature is inconsistent with regard to reporting the prevalence of glenoid bone defects associated with recurrent anterior shoulder instability. This is especially true in cases of larger defects that will ultimately require grafting procedures. As described by Piasecki et al. [5], this may be due in part to underreporting of these defects as a result of a lack of a uniform way to actually evaluate the glenoid rim for defects following an instability event. Nevertheless, as described by Taylor and Arciero [6], glenoid bone defects can be seen in up to 22 % of first time, traumatic dislocators. With regard to the actual rate of glenoid defects in cases of recurrent instability, the literature is varied, with reports ranging from 0 to 90 % [3, 7–10] however, as elegantly noted by Sugaya et al. [10], there is likely some degree of glenoid bone loss in the majority of patients presenting recurrent instability. Finally, in patients with failed prior surgical stabilization procedures, the rate of associated glenoid bone deficiency has been reported as high as 89 % [11].

6.3   Natural History of Glenoid Bone Defects

The natural history of glenoid bone defects associated with instability events remains unknown. While there is certainly a strong association between the existence of glenoid bone deficiency and recurrent anterior shoulder instability events, it is unclear as to how these lesions evolve over time, and more importantly, the clinical implications of these defects remains unknown. For example, some patients may sustain a glenoid bone defect at the time of their initial instability event [12, 13] but may remain asymptomatic in the future, and thus the progression of the defect over time (or lack thereof) will remain unknown. Other patients, however, may sustain a similar lesion at the time of their initial instability event but may become symptomatic in the future with recurrent instability episodes. In these cases, the bony defects have been shown to undergo progression, erosion, or remodeling over time. For example, Mologne et al. [14] reported an attritional pattern to these bony defects in a series of patients approximately 15 months after initial instability event. In this series, nearly 50 % of the glenoids demonstrated erosive bone loss *without* any identifiable glenoid fracture fragment. Other authors have shown that in cases of chronic instability as well as in cases of rim defects, resorption occurs over time [7, 15].

6.4   Pathoanatomy and Biomechanics

The glenohumeral joint allows for more unrestricted range of motion than any other joint in the body. As such, the static and dynamic stabilizers as previously described are critical for containing the congruency of the humeral head articular surface and the glenoid articular surface in order to prevent sublxuation and/or dislocation events [10, 16]. Loss of bone in the anteroinferior glenoid therefore creates a mismatch between the glenoid and humerus as the available articular arc is reduced. It is this articular arc, or the glenoid articular surface and its inherent concavity, that contain the humeral head and prevent excessive translation. Further, a reduced articular arc as caused by a glenoid bony defect reduces the surface area of the glenoid and makes it more difficult to resist axial forces. This inability to withstand normal axial loading forces thus increases the relative shear forces distributed to the capsulolabral complex, which can be problematic in the setting of Bankart repair and/or capsular plication [11]. With such defects, the depth of the articular conformity is decreased as the normal concavity-compression restraint to anterior instability is diminished. This can be especially problematic in cases of concomitant humeral head Hill-Sachs lesions, particularly in cases of tracking lesions [17–19].

6.5   Mechanism

While the mechanism of acute anterior shoulder instability is well-understood, the cause of glenoid bone defects is less well-defined. The mechanism of injury in these cases is likely multifactorial, and certainly differs depending on whether the injury is acute or chronic upon presentation. Acute glenoid bone defects are likely the result of a direct traumatic event with a substantial axial load imparted on the glenoid [11]. In these cases, the shoulder is often in the provocative position of abduction and external rotation, but it is likely the axial force that causes the bony injury as opposed to the soft tissue disruption seen in most cases of acute anterior shoulder instability. Chronic glenoid bone defects may have initially occurred as a result of a one-time traumatic event, however often times these patients have recurrent instability and as such, the anterior glenoid undergoes a continuous, erosive process.

6.6   Clinical Presentation: History

Assessment of the patient with a glenoid bone defect should always begin with a thorough, directed history. The clinician must elicit the exact onset of symptoms and whether or not the patient experienced a traumatic instability event. Patients describing an initial high-energy event in which the glenoid is likely to have sustained a substantial axial load may be more likely to have glenoid bone deficiency in addition to soft tissue disruption of the anteroinferior shoulder. Further, patients who report recurrent subluxation or dislocation events after the initial injury are more likely to have lost a portion of the bony constraint that normally stabilizes the glenohumeral joint even in the setting of capsulolabral injury. Patients may specifically complain of a sensation of subluxation with activities at midranges of abduction (20–60°) [19], even with low-energy activities of daily living such as showering or grooming. A major red flag indicating the likelihood of glenoid bone involvement is a progressive ease of subluxation with lower energy activities. The clinician should also ask about prior instability events to both shoulders, as well as generalized joint laxity, as these findings may dictate further work-up. The history must include prior treatment, including prior surgical procedures and rehabilitation protocols, as well as the patient's response to prior to treatment. Finally, the clinician must ask about preinjury activity level and desire to return to sport/work, as this information will certainly play a role on potential treatment options.

6.7   Clinical Presentation: Physical Examination

After a complete history, a focused physical examination of both shoulders should be performed. It may be preferable to begin with the uninjured shoulder in order to establish a baseline for strength, range of motion, and stability. Both shoulders should be visually inspected with the goal of identifying scapular dyskinesia, muscular atrophy, and any evidence of prior surgical scars. Following inspection, the shoulder should be assessed for active and passive range of motion, strength, and sensation. It is especially important to document the strength of the rotator cuff musculature, particularly the subscapularis, in patients who have undergone prior surgery. Provocative testing should be performed last, with an emphasis on labrum testing and instability testing. All maneuvers should be compared to the uninjured shoulder, as patients may have baseline laxity. Patients with clinically significant glenoid bone defects are likely to have positive apprehension tests in the midranges of abduction (20–60°) [19], as compared to patients who have instability without bony involvement. It must be mentioned that the physical examination is helpful in identifying patients with anteroinferior shoulder instability, but may prove difficult in distinguishing those patients with bony defects. Finally, all patients should have a focused examination of the cervical spine in order to rule-out radiating axial pain as a cause for any shoulder complaints.

6.8 Imaging Studies

Imaging studies are quite helpful in the evaluation of patients with suspected anterior glenoid bone defects. Plain radiographs are typically the first study of choice, however this modality is limited in its utility to accurately show or quantify glenoid bone loss. The radiographic series should contain the standard AP, lateral, and axillary views (Fig. 6.1). These images can be useful in picking up larger bony fragments or larger glenoid articular arc defects. The glenoid profile view can also be helpful in this setting [7, 20]. Specialized views including the apical oblique and West Point views [21–23] are especially helpful as they are taken at a projection angled relative to the glenoid face (as opposed to the previously mentioned views, which are more parallel to the glenoid face). Further, the Stryker notch view

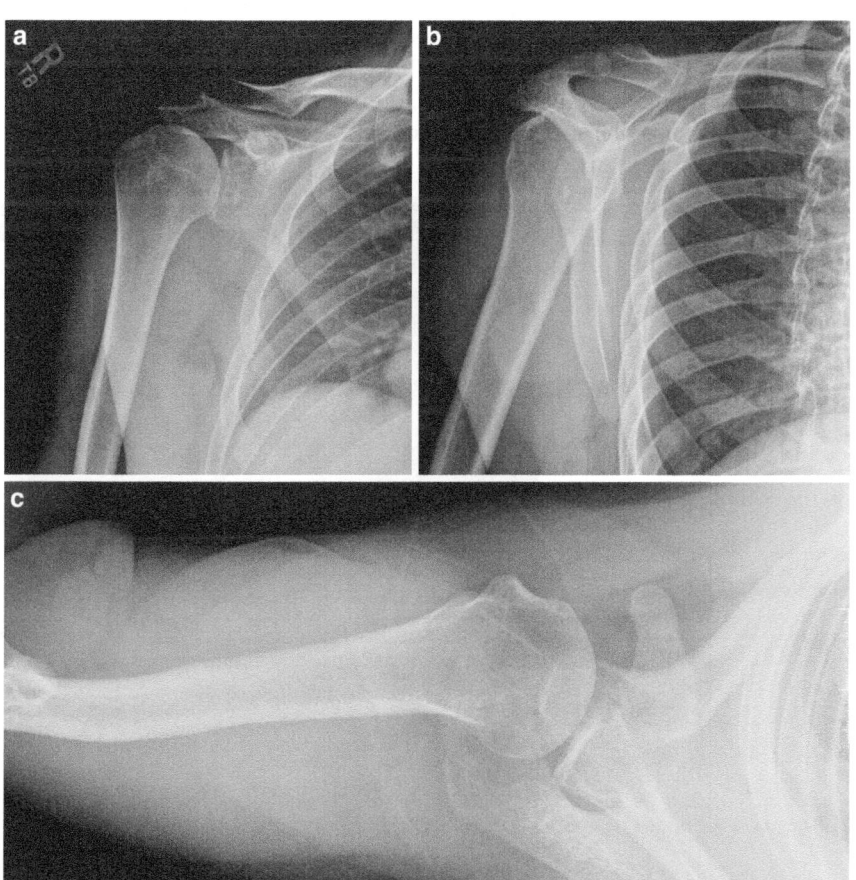

Fig. 6.1 AP, supraspinatous outlet, and axillary radiographs of the right shoulder in a patient with a small (<15 %) anterior glenoid bone defect

is helpful in elucidating associated Hill-Sachs defects on the humeral head, which are important to identify as larger defects may alter the intended surgical plan [24].

While radiographs are helpful, the imaging modality of choice for assessing glenoid bony defects is computed tomography (CT) (Fig. 6.2). Not only can CT identify the morphology of the bony defect and the impact the fracture has on glenoid articular arc, but it can also assist with quantifying the amount of glenoid bone loss, which again has treatment implications. Recent work by Sugaya and Huysmans [10, 25] have elegantly described the morphology of the glenoid rim in the setting of recurrent anterior shoulder instability. With these methods, which utilize conventional and three-dimensional CT scanning, glenoid osseous deficiency can be quantified as a percentage of the normal inferior glenoid surface area. Specifically, a circle is drawn over the inferior two-thirds of the glenoid image, after which any missing bone within the circle is digitally measured and expressed as a percentage of the total surface area of the inferior circle. This method helps for preoperative planning, as the size of the defect, in association with clinical symptoms, often determines the surgical method.

Finally, magnetic resonance imaging (MRI) and/or arthrography (MRA) can be used to evaluate the joint as well as any soft tissue injuries. These modalities are helpful in planning the capsulolabral portion of surgical repair as well as for

Fig. 6.2 Preoperative 3D CT scan of the right shoulder demonstrating a large (>25 %) anterior glenoid bone defect

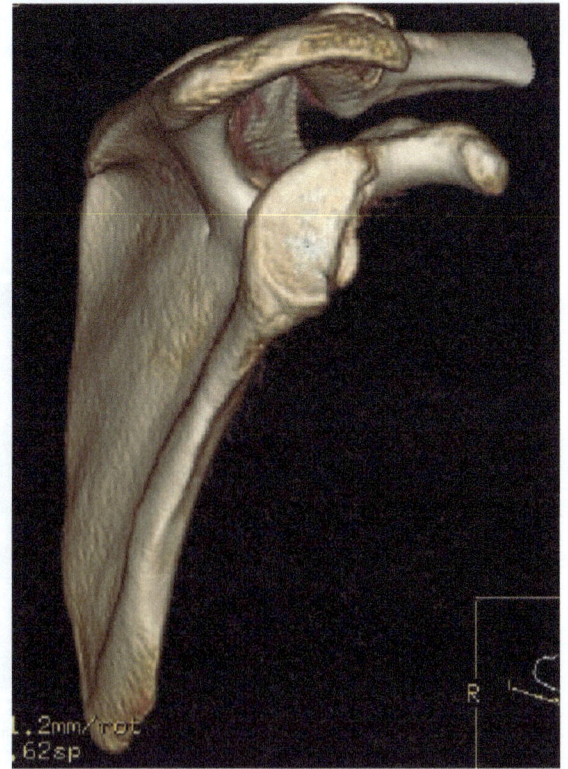

identifying articular surface cartilaginous lesions. Nevertheless, CT remains the study of choice for quantifying anterior glenoid bone defects.

6.9   Diagnostic Arthroscopy

In addition to CT, diagnostic arthroscopy is well-described with regard to its ability to accurately describe glenoid bone loss in the setting of anterior shoulder instability (Fig. 6.3). Direct visualization of the bony defect with arthroscopy gives the surgeon a real-time assessment of the morphology of the glenoid articular rim as well as allows for the assessment of surrounding osseous and soft tissue structures, which is of utmost importance in planning the potential fixation technique. As demonstrated in a cadaveric study by Huysmans et al. [25], the normal inferior glenoid is bounded by a nearly perfect circle [26–28] Inside this circle is the well-described "bare spot" which has been shown to mark the center of the circle. As described by Lo and colleagues, the bare spot can be used arthroscopically to quantify glenoid bone loss. When the arthroscope is in the anterosuperior portal, a calibrated probe can be inserted through the posterior portal to measure the anterior-posterior width of the defect at the level of the bare spot. This is accomplished by measuring the distance from the anterior and posterior rims to the bare spot. Given the theory of the inferior glenoid shape as a perfect circle, when the anterior measurement is less than the posterior measurement, anterior bone loss is confirmed. The amount of bone loss can then be quantified and expressed as a percentage of the diameter of the normal inferior glenoid by assuming that the normal inferior glenoid diameter is twice the distance from the posterior glenoid rim to the bare spot. As will be discussed in the next section, this number, or

Fig. 6.3 Arthroscopic image demonstrating the osseous defect on the anterior glenoid rim

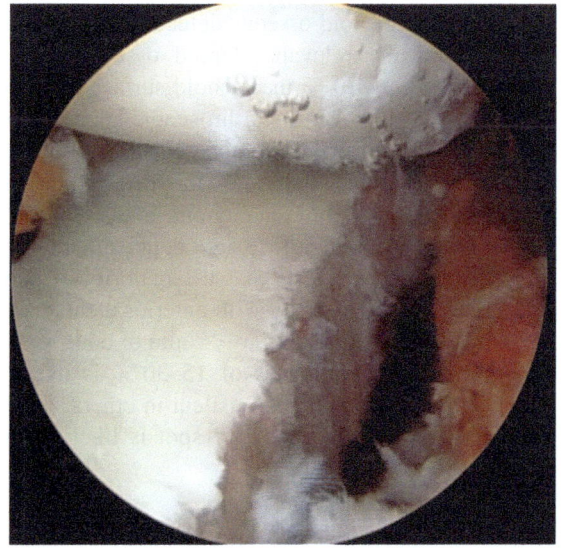

percentage of glenoid bone loss, is extremely relevant when it comes to selecting the most appropriate treatment option. As is evident, anterior glenoid osseous defects disrupt the normal perfect circle morphology of the inferior glenoid, leading to the description of a glenoid with such a defect as an "inverted pear" [9–11, 14, 29].

6.10   Clinically Relevant Glenoid Bone Loss: The Critical Limit

While both CT and diagnostic arthroscopy can effectively quantify the amount of glenoid osseous deficiency in patients with anterior shoulder instability, the determination of precisely how much bone loss is truly clinically relevant is actually more important. For example, if a patient is found incidentally to have a significant amount of glenoid bone loss as determined by CT, yet he or she is completely asymptomatic, then the ability to quantify the defect becomes irrelevant.

Multiple authors have attempted to biomechanically determine the "critical limit" at which glenoid bone deficiency clinically destabilizes the glenohumeral joint [5]. Itoi et al. [16] analyzed the peak forces required to cause humeral head translation on the glenoid with sequentially larger glenoid osseous defects. The degree of glenoid bone defect was quantified by the width of each resection as a percentage of the total width of the glenoid, which translated to 9, 21, 34, and 46 %. As could be inferred, glenohumeral stability decreased (less force required for translation) as the degree of bone loss increased, with a notable drop off at defects ≥ 21 % (corresponding to average defect width of 6.8 mm). Of note, this study was performed with the glenoid osteotomies made at a 45° inclination to the long axis of the glenoid, as opposed to straight anterior-posterior. In a similar biomechanical study, Greis et al. [30]. reported increased glenohumeral contact pressures with glenoid osseous defects >30 %. Thus, these biomechanical studies suggest clinically relevant glenoid osseous defects occur when the lesion is approximately 21–30 % the glenoid surface area (corresponding to 6–7 mm).

As described above, the arthroscopic appearance of the glenoid as an inverted pear when viewed from the anterosuperior portal is associated with clinical glenohumeral instability. In the lab, this inverted pear appearance has been shown to occur with a mean anterior glenoid bone loss of 7.5 mm, which corresponds to 28 % of total glenoid surface area deficiency at the level of the bare spot [9, 11]. Overall, the data suggests that the majority of patients will have clinically significant shoulder instability with anterior glenoid width loss >30 % at the level of the bare spot, corresponding to <4 mm of bone remaining anterior to the bare spot. Anterior glenoid width loss of 15–30 % is likely to cause symptoms in some patients, but may be clinically silent in others. Finally, anterior glenoid width loss <15 % at the level of the bare spot is likely to be asymptomatic in nearly all patients [5, 31, 32].

While these numbers are commonly referenced, it is critical that the orthopaedic surgeon fully evaluate each patient on an individual basis, as some patients may remain clinically stable with substantial defects while others may experience recurrent subluxation with lesions that would otherwise appear quantitatively irrelevant This is especially true in patients with concomitant humeral head bone defects, especially engaging Hill-Sachs defects [24].

6.11   Nonoperative Treatment

The use of nonoperative treatment strategies for glenoid bone defects in the setting of anterior shoulder instability depends on the size of the defect and the patient [5]. While it is always helpful to strengthen the dynamic stabilizers of the shoulder joint, including the periscapular and rotator cuff musculature, therapy alone cannot address the instability that occurs when the static stabilizers of the shoulder are disrupted, especially with large bone defects. Similarly, common non-operative modalities including bracing, ice, anti-inflammatories, and corticosteroid injections may help to control pain, but are clearly unlikely to improve recurrent instability symptoms in a patient with a significant disrupted glenoid articular arc. As the degree of bone loss increases, the congruency of the humeral head on the glenoid decreases, and as described in detail above, recurrent instability is likely to worsen with increasing ease of subsequent instability events. Thus, patient activity level (in particular their likelihood to engage in activities that will load the shoulder joint) as well as defect size, are the two factors most likely to influence the decision for surgical intervention.

Patients who may benefit from non-operative treatment strategies are older, lower-demand individuals with smaller sized defects (i.e., <15 %). Patients who are voluntary subluxators, medically unfit for surgery, who are unwilling to comply with rehabilitation protocols, who have unrealistic postoperative expectations are also better candidates for nonsurgical management.

Nonoperative treatment strategies typically involve an acute period of immoblization followed by strict rehabilitation under the guidance of a therapist familiar with scapular stabilizing exercises. Currently, there is debate over whether immoblization in the standard internal rotation position versus external rotation is more beneficial in decreasing the risk of recurrent instability events [33, 34].

6.12   Operative Treatment (by Amounts of Bone Loss, with Outcomes)

Surgical intervention for patients with recurrent shoulder instability associated with glenoid bone loss varies by the size of the defect as well as by other patient specific factors, including age, degree of concomitant injuries, and activity level. An algorithmic approach [5, 32] has been proposed and is useful as a guide for

Table 6.1 Surgical options for glenoid bone loss

< 15 % bone loss*	No specific surgical procedure needed for the glenoid bone loss

15–25 % bone loss*	Low Demand Athlete
	• Soft tissue stabilization with bone fragment incorporation
	High Demand Athlete
	• Soft tissue stabilization **with:**
	• Open versus Arthroscopic[#] bony fragment fixation
	  if glenoid fragment available) **OR:**
	Glenoid augmentation with Latarjet, ICBG, or allograft
	  reconstruction (distal tibia or glenoid) (if glenoid
	  fragment not available)

>25 % bone loss*	• Soft tissue stabilization with:
	• Open versus Arthroscopic[#] bony fragment fixation
	  (if glenoid fragment **OR:**
	Glenoid augmentation with Latarjet, ICBG, or allograft
	  reconstruction (distal tibia or glenoid) (if glenoid
	  fragment not available)

*Must quantify glenoid bone loss via preoperative 3D CT and/or diagnostic arthroscopy prior to treatment decision
[#]Must use caution with Arthroscopic procedures given technical demands with larger bony defects

surgical planning (Table 6.1), however, there are many factors to take into account including patient activity level and postoperative demands. The majority of patients with this injury are indicated for surgery should an initial course of nonoperative treatment prove ineffective. Further, many authors would advocate for surgery in young, first-time dislocators, given the high rate of recurrent anterior shoulder instability in this specific patient population [8, 11]. The same can be said for patients who are extremely active in overhead and/or contact activities as well as those with large defects (>30 %) at the time of initial diagnosis. It must be emphasized that operative treatment for patients with anterior shoulder instability does not always include treatment of the glenoid bony defect, especially in cases of smaller defects (<15 %), in which sound treatment of the soft tissue capsulolabral defects is likely adequate treatment.

6.12.1 Bone Loss <15 %

Surgical options for bony defects <15 % include soft tissue stabilization only (no treatment of the osseous defect), direct anatomic repair, and arthroscopic repair with suture anchors. Some authors have shown that surgical fixation of even small defects has a positive effect on clinical outcomes. Bigliani [7] described a series of 22 patients found to have small avulsion-type fractures of the glenoid rim in the setting of recurrent anterior instability after an initial traumatic event. The majority of these fractures were treated with direct open anatomic repair of the capsulolabral tissue with the bony fragment to the glenoid rim. At 2.5 years following surgery,

86 % of patients were satisfied, with 72 % experiencing normal shoulder stability. The authors reported 94 % of the patients who underwent fracture repair remained stable postoperatively, while 40 % of the patients who did not receive fracture repair experienced recurrent instability. Porcellini et al. [12] described a series of 25 patients with acute glenoid rim avulsion fractures approximately 2 years following arthroscopic stabilization with suture anchor fixation of the bony fragment to the labral interface. At follow-up, 92 % of patients had returned to their previous level of activity/sport.

As described, the majority of patients with recurrent anterior shoulder instability will have some degree of anterior glenoid osseous deficiency in addition to the Bankart lesion. In these cases, for the reasons mentioned above, the relatively small glenoid defect is unlikely to be responsible for the recurrent instability events as the degree of bone loss anterior to the bare spot is minimal, and thus unlikely to be clinically relevant. Thus, in these cases, while a minimum "critical value" of anterior glenoid osseous deficiency has not yet been clinically established, it can be inferred form the work of Itoi [16] as well as the studies by Sugaya [10] that such small defects are unlikely to require surgical correction.

6.12.2 Bone Loss 15–30 %

As the degree of glenoid rim osseous insufficiency grows, the likelihood of that defect being clinically significant also grows. Surgical options for defects larger than 15 % but smaller than 25–30 % are more varied, and can include soft tissue stabilization only, arthroscopic stabilization (Figs. 6.4 and 6.5) with bone fragment incorporation, the Latarjet Procedure, as well as autograft augmentation for glenoid reconstruction. A variety of factors should be carefully considered when deciding amongst these treatment options, including availability of the bone fragment, patient-specific shoulder demands (high versus low demand), and again, size of the defect.

Sugaya et al. [15] have demonstrated excellent clinical outcomes following arthroscopic reduction and suture anchor fixation of glenoid rim avulsion fractures averaging 24.5 % of the inferior glenoid surface. All 42 patients in this series had documented glenoid bone deficiency and had experienced at least 6 months of recurrent instability. At an average 34 months postoperatively, 93 % of patients had good–excellent Rowe and UCLA scores and 95 % of patients returned to sport. Interestingly, 12 patients underwent CT scan at final follow-up and in all cases, bony union of the glenoid fracture fragment to the glenoid rim was demonstrated. Similarly, Mologne et al. [14] reported on the outcomes of 23 patients with documented glenoid bone deficiency and recurrent anterior instability at a mean 34 months following arthroscopic stabilization. In this series, the average bony defect size ranged from 20–30 % width loss. At follow-up, an overall 14.2 % failure rate was reported, however these failures were all within the group of patients who had not undergone incorporation of the fracture fragment into the repair due to unavailability of the fracture fragment.

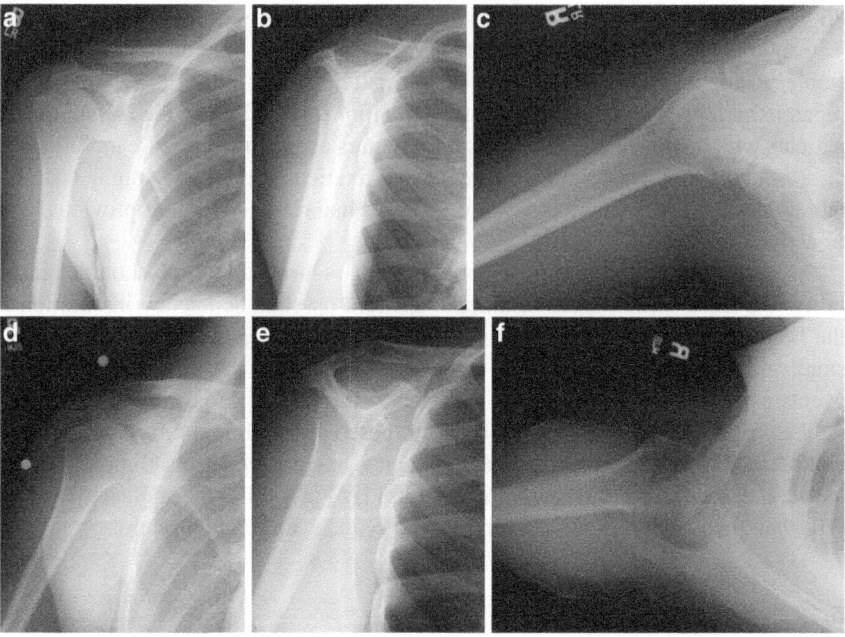

Fig. 6.4 Pre and postoperative radiographs (AP, supraspinatous outlet, and axillary) of the right shoulder demonstrating direct suture repair of a glenoid bone fragment

The surgical decision-making becomes more complex as both patient-specific demands increase as well as the size of the bony defect. Burkhart and DeBeer [11] reported an 89 % failure rate of soft-tissue only (no bony fragment incorporation) stabilization in high-level contact athletes with anterior shoulder instability and defect sizes of approximately 25–30 %. Thus, as described above, for these larger defects, the surgeon should attempt to incorporate the fracture fragment into the soft tissue repair for optimal joint stabilization. If and when the fracture fragment is not available for fixation (due to erosion, attrition, etc.), and the defect is thought to be clinically significant, surgical augmentation of the glenoid via an open procedure with autograft or allograft must be considered. These are some of the most challenging clinical scenarios, as in these patients, it is not always clear if the defect is clinically relevant as it is too small to be considered a "must-fix" fragment while it is also too big to simply be ignored. The surgeon must therefore balance the risk of recurrent instability if a soft tissue only repair is performed with the complications associated with open glenoid bone augmentation.

6.12.3 Bone Loss >30 %

Significant bony defects of the glenoid rim almost always require a surgical approach involving glenoid bone augmentation. As noted above, glenoid osseous

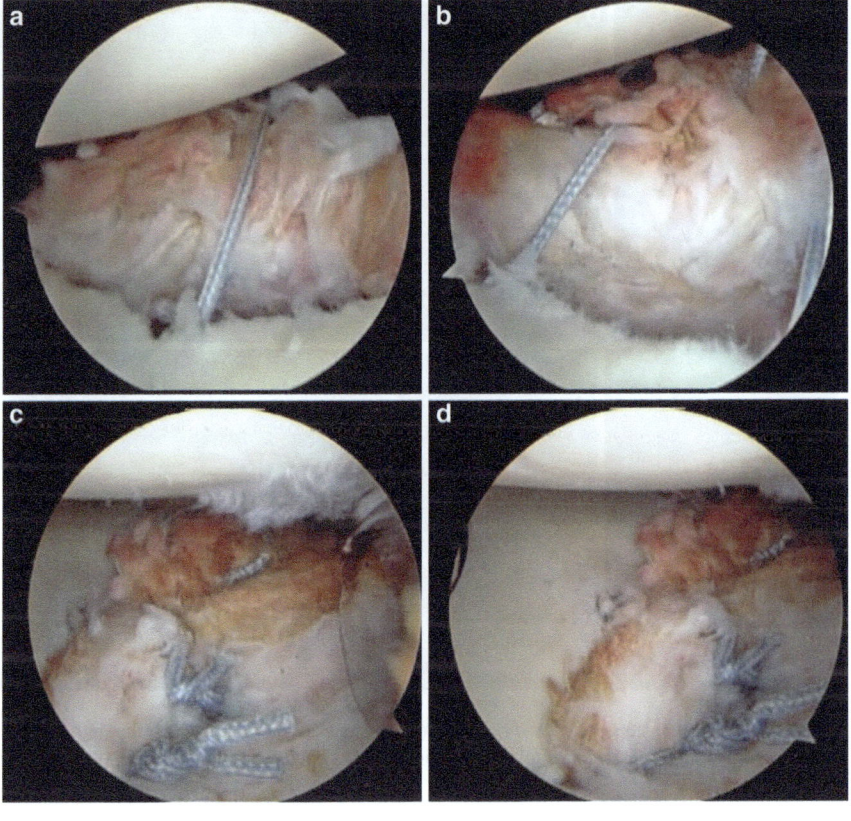

Fig. 6.5 Arthroscopic images demonstrating the use of direct suture repair of a glenoid bone defect onto the anterior glenoid rim; also visible is the antero-inferior labrum and the repaired fragment-labrum interface

deficiency of >25–30 % of the anterior glenoid width at the level of the bare spot is equivalent to a significantly reduced amount of bone stock anterior to the bare spot, typically <4–5 mm. These are the defects that cause an inverted pear appearance of the glenoid surface when viewed from the anterosuperior portal arthroscopically. The goals of surgery are thus to improve glenohumeral stability by restoring the glenoid rim articular arc [16, 35].

In the acute setting, it may be possible to directly repair the fracture fragment with the capsulolabral tissue back to the anteroinferior glenoid rim. The key for this type of procedure is anatomic reduction of the fracture fragment and anatomic reconstruction of the glenoid articular arc. Such an approach typically requires an open procedure with suture anchors and/or screw fixation, and medium-term outcomes have been encouraging [36]. Anecdotal reports of arthroscopic fracture fragment reduction followed by percutaneous screw fixation have been described, however additional, longer-term studies are needed before definitive recommendations on this treatment option can be made.

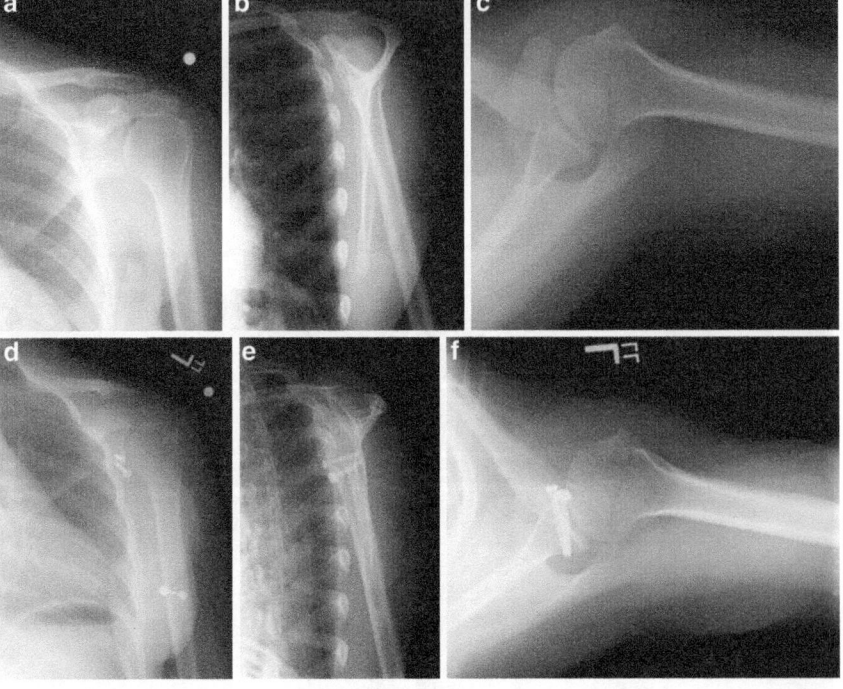

Fig. 6.6 Pre and postoperative radiographs (AP, lateral, and axillary) of the left shoulder demonstrating Latarjet fixation of a large anterior glenoid bone defect; visible is the interference screw fixation technique

While direct fracture fragment fixation has been reported, glenoid bone augmentation is the more commonly employed approach for significant glenoid bony defects. Often, the avulsed glenoid fragment is missing (attritional loss) or is too small (resorption) to allow for direct screw fixation. Further, the remaining glenoid rim is often highly attenuated due to recurrent instability events, and so even in the case of an existing fracture fragment big enough for fixation, the glenoid rim morphology is so destroyed that anatomic reconstruction is impossible.

Multiple techniques for glenoid bone augmentation have been described, and currently there is no "gold standard". Both autograft and allograft techniques have been reported with acceptable outcomes. The key to all of the approaches is to achieve anatomic restoration of the glenoid rim in order to adequately restore the articular contact surface with the humeral head. Surgeon experience and preference thus often dictate the procedure of choice.

The most common approach to glenoid augmentation in the setting of anterior glenohumeral instability with glenoid osseous defects >25–30 % involves transfer of the coracoid process to the anteroinferior glenoid rim, known as the Latarjet or Bristow procedure (Fig. 6.6) [37–41]. First described in 1958 by Helfet, this procedure involve transfer of the coracoid process with its attached conjoined tendon (short head of biceps, coracobrachialis) to the anterior surface of the gle-noid. The Latarjet procedure is preferred to the traditional Bristow procedure as the Latarjet uses a longer segment of coracoid, fixing its long axis in parallel to the glenoid rim, as opposed to the Bristow procedure in which the glenoid is fixed in a perpendicular position.

With regard to technique, the procedure is typically performed via an open, anterior approach. The pectoralis minor tendon is released, revealing the coracoid process. The coracoid is then osteotomized proximal to its angle, rotated 90°, passed through a split the subscapularis tendon, and positioned on the anteroinferior gle-noid. A variety of fixation methods have been described; typically two 3.5 mm metal screws are used to fix the coracoid graft in position as flush as possible with the native glenoid. Minor adjustments can be made to the graft with a burr in an attempt to keep it flush with the glenoid. Some surgeons leave a remnant of the coracoa-cromial ligament attached to the coracoid to act as a soft tissue stump for direct repair of the capsulolabral tissue to the graft. The native capsule is fixed posterior to the coracoid graft with suture anchors or bone tunnels, making the graft an extra-articular extension of the articular arc of the glenoid. Alternatively, the capsule can be repaired to the anterior aspect of the coracoid so that the graft in intra-articular.

This procedure improves shoulder stability in several ways. First, the graft itself increases the glenoid contact surface area and thus increases the available articular arc for the humeral head to rotate on prior to subluxation. Next, the conjoined tendon acts as a dynamic buttress across the anteroinferior glenoid to limit anterior humeral head translation when the shoulder is in the abduction-externally rotated position. Finally, graft and conjoined tendon create a tenodesis effect as they are passed through the subscapularis tendon, which further reinforces a redundant anteroinferior capsule. Many modifications of the Bristow-Latarjet procedure have been described with encouraging outcomes; one variation involves releasing the graft from all soft tissue and using it as a free bone block.

Outcomes for the Latarjet procedure and its modifications have been encour-aging. Hovelius et al. [37, 38] prospectively described the outcomes following Bristow-Latarjet stabilization in 118 patients with recurrent anterior shoulder instability at an average 15.2 years following surgery. The authors reported a redislocation rate of 3.4 % and a recurrent subluxation rate of 10 %, with good–excellent outcomes as determined by the Rowe score in 86 %. In a separate report, the authors described the occurrence of postoperative glenohumeral arthropathy (mild in 35 %, moderate-severe in 14 %) in this same cohort and noted increased frequency in patients whose grafts were placed at or lateral to the glenoid. Another study by Hovelius compared the outcomes following Bristow-Latarjet to a retro-spective cohort of patients undergoing soft-tissue stabilization and found similar rates of recurrance, arthropathy, and overall patient satisfaction [39]. Longer-term outcomes at 26 years following Bristow-Latarjet have been described [41], how-ever there are concerns regarding the development of stiffness, especially in the plane of external rotation [39].

All-arthroscopic Latarjet techniques [42–44] have recently been described. First described by Lafosse and colleagues, this minimally-invasive technique involves exposure, coracoid preparation, coracoid drilling and osteotomy, coracoid transfer, and coracoid fixation. Given the improved visibility with this procedure via the use of arthroscopy, in theory it is easier to avoid anterior overhand of the bone-block once fixed. As overhang is linked to the development of postoperative arthropathy, the potential advantage of arthroscopic Latarjet as compared to the open technique is obvious. Nevertheless, this procedure is technically demanding even for the most experienced of arthroscopists, and so its use is not yet widespread. Early outcomes reported by Lafosse [42] have been encouraging, with 91 of 100 patients reporting excellent outcomes scores at an average 26 months following arthroscopic Latarjet; further, 69 % of patients had no evidence of arthrosis at final follow-up.

Bony augmentation with iliac crest (autograft and allograft) has also been described. The bony contour of the iliac crest is similar geometrically compared to the glenoid rim, making anatomic fixation possible. Technically, after iliac crest harvest (or preparation if using allograft), the curve of the inner table of the iliac wing is matched to that of the glenoid, with the concave inner surface facing laterally and the cancellous base of the graft secured with screws to the glenoid neck. Ideally, the natural contour of the iliac wing matches that of the glenoid articular arc. Following fixation with screws, the anteroinferior capsule is secured to the bone block so that the block can be intra or extra-articular.

Similar to the Latarjet, satisfactory clinical outcomes have been reported following iliac crest glenoid augmentation. Haaker et al. [45] reported the outcomes of 24 patients undergoing iliac crest autograft at an average 42 months following surgery; no patients had recurrent instability and 90 % were satisfied with the procedure. Warner et al. [19] also reported on the outcomes following iliac crest autograft in 11 patients with recurrent anterior instability. At an average 33 months following surgery, there were no episodes of recurrent instability.

The use of allograft tissue for the treatment of large glenoid bone defects in the setting of recurrent anterior shoulder instability has been described [5, 31, 32]. Allografts clearly eliminate the potential morbidity of using autograft tissue and allow the surgeon to match the donor tissue to the exact geometry of the bony defect, however the use of allografts also has certain inherent pitfalls, including the risk of disease transmission, failure to incorporate, and cost. Reports of fresh osteochondral glenoid, frozen humeral head, frozen femoral head, and fresh distal tibial osteochondral allograft have all been reported, however to date, no short or long-term outcomes studies are available. While fresh glenoid allograft would intuitively seem to make the most sense, these grafts are difficult to obtain for a variety of reasons, including graft contamination and availability.

Interestingly, the anatomy of the distal tibia makes it an excellent theoretical graft option for glenoid bone defects [5, 32, 46]. The lateral aspect of the distal tibia has a near identical radius of curvature with that of the glenoid and is composed of dense, corticocancelleous bone (Fig. 6.7). Similarly, the glenoid and tibial cartilage thickness are also very similar, allowing the graft to recreate the anatomy of the missing glenoid. The technique for glenoid augmentation has been described in detail in several recent reports (Figs. 6.8, 6.9, 6.10). In brief, a standard deltopectoral approach is used with exposure of the glenohumeral joint.

Fig. 6.7 Photograph demonstrating the near "perfect fit" with regard to the radius of curvature of the lateral aspect of the distal tibia with that of the glenoid surface

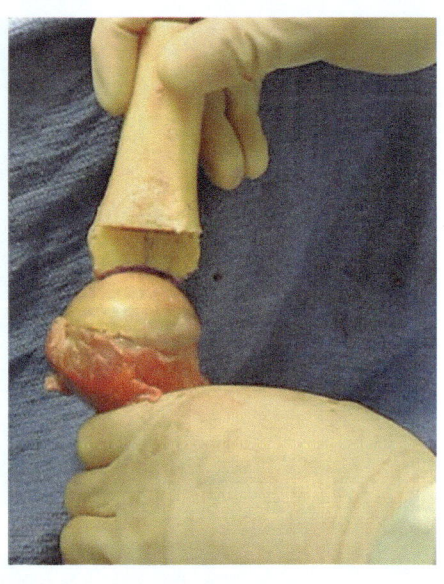

During preparation of the glenoid surface, it is important to preserve as much labrum as possible for further repair. The distal tibial allograft is prepared separately, using the lateral aspect of the tibial plafond and size-matching the graft to the width of the glenoid defect. The graft depth must but cut to allow sufficient subchondral bone to allow screw fixation to the glenoid. The graft is then fixed temporarily to the glenoid with two 1.6 mm Kirschner wires placed at a 45° angle to the articular surface and then secured with 3.5 mm fully threaded cortical screws that are placed as parallel to the glenoid face as possible. The capsulolabral complex is then repaired and the screws are tightened, followed by wound closure. Initial case reports do show encouraging results with this procedure, however larger, longer-term are needed before definitive conclusions can be made.

6.13   Summary

Glenoid bone defects in the setting of recurrent anterior shoulder instability can be difficult to treat. Defects are often unrecognized until the time of surgery, and it can be difficult to determine which lesions are truly contributing to symptomatic instability. An intact glenoid articular arc is crucial for a stable articulation with the humeral head, and loss of articular congruency can prove detrimental in recurrent anterior shoulder instability. Preoperative evaluation with CT followed by diagnostic arthroscopy when indicated is necessary to determine the size of the defect. The size of the defect, coupled with patient-specific factors including activity level, are major factors in determining appropriate treatment options. In general, defects <15 % of the glenoid width can be treated with soft tissue

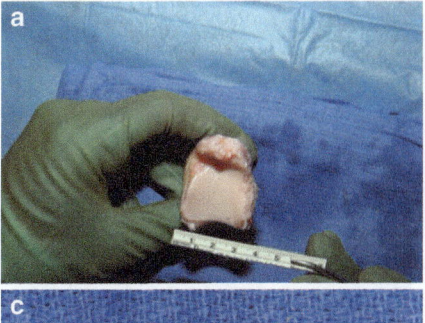
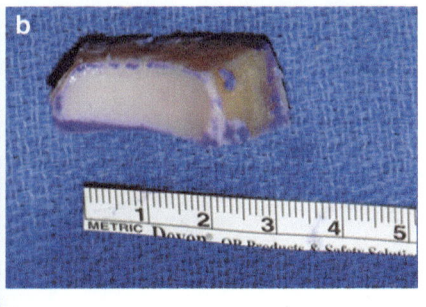
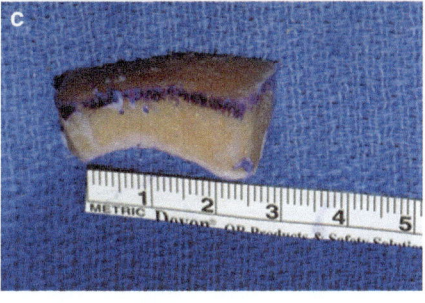

Fig. 6.8 Intraoperative photographs demonstrating measurements of the distal tibial allograft; as shown in biomechanical laboratory work, the lateral aspect of the distal tibia is a near "perfect fit" to the anatomy of the glenoid with regard to radius of curvature, glenoid and tibial cartilage thickness, and the density of the corticocancellous bone

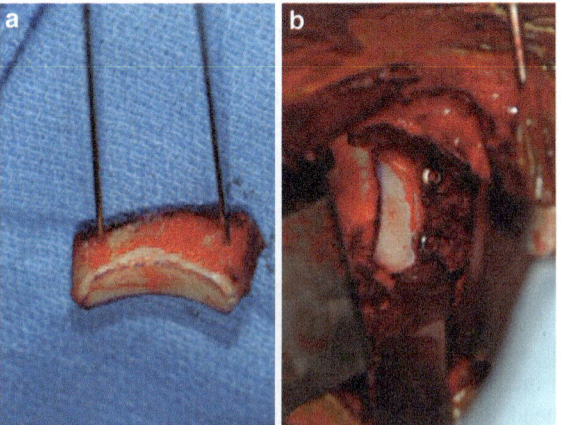

Fig. 6.9 Intraoperative photographs demonstrating the use of the distal tibial allograft technique for reconstruction of large anterior glenoid bone defects. Following appropriate size-matching (see Fig. 6.8), the tibial allograft is cut in such a way that allows enough depth of subchondral bone to permit placement of 3.5 mm screws to secure the graft to the glenoid. To secure the graft, two 1.5 mm Kirshner wires are placed at a 45° angle to the articular surface of the graft. For the actual fixation contruct, as mentioned, two 3.5 mm screws are used to secure the graft

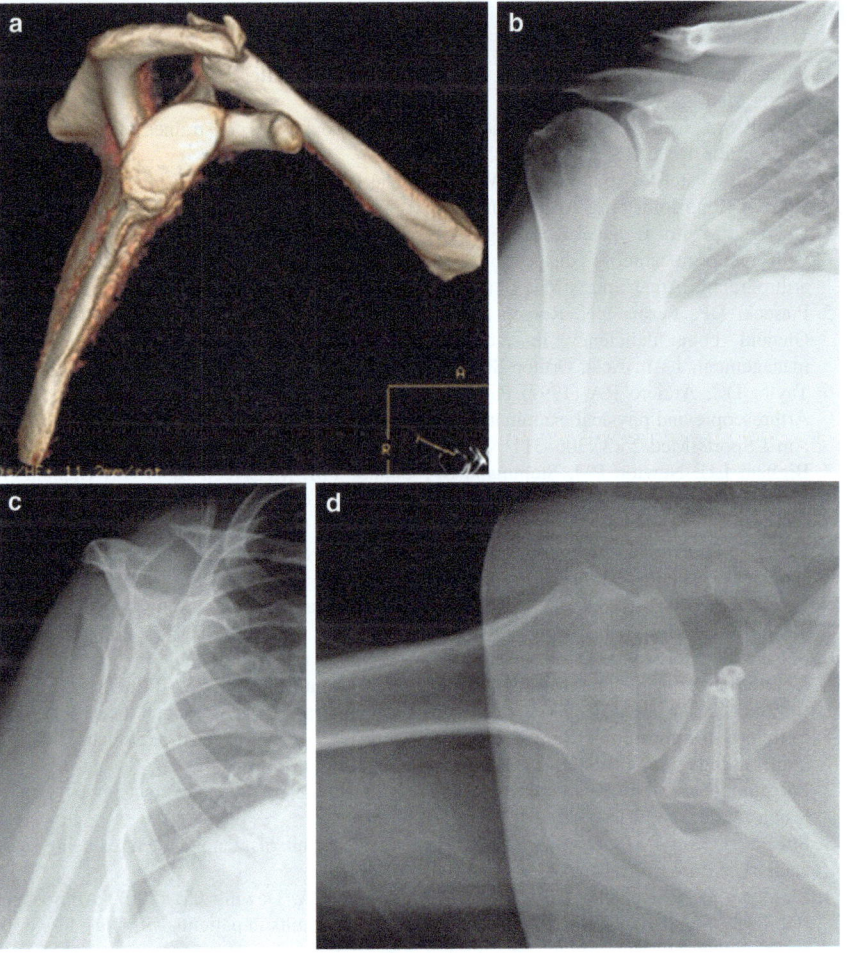

Fig. 6.10 Pre and postoperative images of the right shoulder with a large anterior glenoid bone defect; postoperative radiographs demonstrate appropriate placement of a distal tibial allograft construct for glenoid reconstruction

stabilization alone while defects >30 % of the glenoid width often require autograft or allograft glenoid augmentation. Defects between 15–30 % are in an indeterminate zone, and attention must be paid to the size of the defect and the demands of the patients. In general, patients in this group can be treated with direct fragment repair either through open or arthroscopic techniques as well as glenoid bone autograft or allograft augmentation. With appropriate patient selection criteria and sound surgical technique, the majority of patients with recurrent anterior shoulder instability associated with a glenoid osseous defect can be effectively treated and returned to a high level of function without recurrent instability.

References

1. Hintermann B, Gachter A (1995) Arthroscopic findings after shoulder dislocation. Am J Sports Med 23(5):545–551
2. Howell SM, Galinat BJ (1989) The glenoid-labral socket. A constrained articular surface. Clin Orthop Relat Res 243:122–125
3. Rowe CR, Patel D, Southmayd WW (1978) The Bankart procedure: a long-term end-result study. J Bone Joint Surg Am 60(1):1–16
4. Urayama M, Itoi E, Sashi R, Minagawa H, Sato K (2003) Capsular elongation in shoulders with recurrent anterior dislocation. Quantitative assessment with magnetic resonance arthrography. Am J Sports Med 31(1):64–67
5. Piasecki DP, Verma NN, Romeo AA, Levine WN, Bach BR Jr, Provencher MT (2009) Glenoid bone deficiency in recurrent anterior shoulder instability: diagnosis and management. J Am Acad Orthop Surg 17(8):482–493
6. Taylor DC, Arciero RA (1997) Pathologic changes associated with shoulder dislocations. Arthroscopic and physical examination findings in first-time, traumatic anterior dislocations. Am J Sports Med 25(3):306–311
7. Bigliani LU, Newton PM, Steinmann SP, Connor PM, McLlveen SJ (1998) Glenoid rim lesions associated with recurrent anterior dislocation of the shoulder. Am J Sports Med 26(1):41–45
8. Hovelius L, Eriksson K, Fredin H et al (1983) Recurrences after initial dislocation of the shoulder. Results of a prospective study of treatment. J Bone Joint Surg Am 65(3):343–349
9. Lo IK, Parten PM, Burkhart SS (2004) The inverted pear glenoid: an indicator of significant glenoid bone loss. Arthroscopy 20(2):169–174
10. Sugaya H, Moriishi J, Dohi M, Kon Y, Tsuchiya A (2003) Glenoid rim morphology in recurrent anterior glenohumeral instability. J Bone Joint Surg Am 85-A(5):878–884
11. Burkhart SS, De Beer JF (2000) Traumatic glenohumeral bone defects and their relationship to failure of arthroscopic Bankart repairs: significance of the inverted-pear glenoid and the humeral engaging Hill-Sachs lesion. Arthroscopy 16(7):677–694
12. Porcellini G, Campi F, Paladini P (2002) Arthroscopic approach to acute bony Bankart lesion. Arthroscopy 18(7):764–769
13. Sugaya H, Kon Y, Tsuchiya A (2005) Arthroscopic repair of glenoid fractures using suture anchors. Arthroscopy 21(5):635
14. Mologne TS, Provencher MT, Menzel KA, Vachon TA, Dewing CB (2007) Arthroscopic stabilization in patients with an inverted pear glenoid: results in patients with bone loss of the anterior glenoid. Am J Sports Med 35(8):1276–1283
15. Sugaya H, Moriishi J, Kanisawa I, Tsuchiya A (2005) Arthroscopic osseous Bankart repair for chronic recurrent traumatic anterior glenohumeral instability. J Bone Joint Surg Am 87(8):1752–1760
16. Itoi E, Lee SB, Berglund LJ, Berge LL, An KN (2000) The effect of a glenoid defect on anteroinferior stability of the shoulder after Bankart repair: a cadaveric study. J Bone Joint Surg Am 82(1):35–46
17. Chen AL, Hunt SA, Hawkins RJ, Zuckerman JD (2005) Management of bone loss associated with recurrent anterior glenohumeral instability. Am J Sports Med 33(6):912–925
18. Lazarus MD, Sidles JA, Harryman DT 2nd, Matsen FA 3rd (1996) Effect of a chondral-labral defect on glenoid concavity and glenohumeral stability. A cadaveric model. J Bone Joint Surg Am 78(1):94–102
19. Warner JJ, Gill TJ, O'Hollerhan JD, Pathare N, Millett PJ (2006) Anatomical glenoid reconstruction for recurrent anterior glenohumeral instability with glenoid deficiency using an autogenous tricortical iliac crest bone graft. Am J Sports Med 34(2):205–212
20. Itoi E, Lee SB, Amrami KK, Wenger DE, An KN (2003) Quantitative assessment of classic anteroinferior bony Bankart lesions by radiography and computed tomography. Am J Sports Med 31(1):112–118

21. Garth WP Jr, Slappey CE, Ochs CW (1984) Roentgenographic demonstration of instability of the shoulder: the apical oblique projection. A technical note. J Bone Joint Surg Am 66(9):1450–1453
22. Pavlov H, Warren RF, Weiss CB Jr, Dines DM (1985) The roentgenographic evaluation of anterior shoulder instability. Clin Orthop Relat Res 194:153–158
23. Rokous JR, Feagin JA, Abbott HG (1972) Modified axillary roentgenogram. A useful adjunct in the diagnosis of recurrent instability of the shoulder. Clin Orthop Relat Res 82:84–86
24. Provencher MT, Frank RM, Leclere LE et al (2012) The Hill-Sachs lesion: diagnosis, classification, and management. J Am Acad Orthop Surg 20(4):242–252
25. Huijsmans PE, Haen PS, Kidd M, Dhert WJ, van der Hulst VP, Willems WJ (2007) Quantification of a glenoid defect with three-dimensional computed tomography and magnetic resonance imaging: a cadaveric study. J Shoulder Elbow Surg 16(6):803–809
26. Burkhart SS (2007) The bare spot of the glenoid. Arthroscopy 23(4):449; author reply 449–450
27. Burkhart SS, Debeer JF, Tehrany AM, Parten PM (2002) Quantifying glenoid bone loss arthroscopically in shoulder instability. Arthroscopy 18(5):488–491
28. Huysmans PE, Haen PS, Kidd M, Dhert WJ, Willems JW (2006) The shape of the inferior part of the glenoid: a cadaveric study. J Shoulder Elbow Surg 15(6):759–763
29. Aigner F, Longato S, Fritsch H, Kralinger F (2004) Anatomical considerations regarding the "bare spot" of the glenoid cavity. Surg Radiol Anat 26(4):308–311
30. Greis PE, Scuderi MG, Mohr A, Bachus KN, Burks RT (2002) Glenohumeral articular contact areas and pressures following labral and osseous injury to the anteroinferior quadrant of the glenoid. J Shoulder Elbow Surg 11(5):442–451
31. Bhatia S, Ghodadra NS, Romeo AA et al (2011) The importance of the recognition and treatment of glenoid bone loss in an athletic population. Sports Health 3(5):435–440
32. Provencher MT, Bhatia S, Ghodadra NS et al (2010) Recurrent shoulder instability: current concepts for evaluation and management of glenoid bone loss. J Bone Joint Surg Am 92(Suppl 2):133–151
33. Itoi E, Hatakeyama Y, Kido T et al (2003) A new method of immobilization after traumatic anterior dislocation of the shoulder: a preliminary study. J Shoulder Elbow Surg 12(5):413–415
34. Itoi E, Hatakeyama Y, Sato T et al (2007) Immobilization in external rotation after shoulder dislocation reduces the risk of recurrence. A randomized controlled trial. J Bone Joint Surg Am 89(10):2124–2131
35. Montgomery WH Jr, Wahl M, Hettrich C, Itoi E, Lippitt SB, Matsen FA 3rd (2005) Anteroinferior bone-grafting can restore stability in osseous glenoid defects. J Bone Joint Surg Am 87(9):1972–1977
36. Scheibel M, Magosch P, Lichtenberg S, Habermeyer P (2004) Open reconstruction of anterior glenoid rim fractures. Knee Surg Sports Traumatol Arthrosc 12(6):568–573
37. Hovelius L, Sandstrom B, Saebo M (2006) One hundred eighteen Bristow-Latarjet repairs for recurrent anterior dislocation of the shoulder prospectively followed for fifteen years: study II-the evolution of dislocation arthropathy. J Shoulder Elbow Surg 15(3):279–289
38. Hovelius L, Sandstrom B, Sundgren K, Saebo M (2004) One hundred eighteen Bristow-Latarjet repairs for recurrent anterior dislocation of the shoulder prospectively followed for fifteen years: study I—clinical results. J Shoulder Elbow Surg 13(5):509–516
39. Hovelius LK, Sandstrom BC, Rosmark DL, Saebo M, Sundgren KH, Malmqvist BG (2001) Long-term results with the Bankart and Bristow-Latarjet procedures: recurrent shoulder instability and arthropathy. J Shoulder Elbow Surg 10(5):445–452
40. Mackenzie DB (1984) The treatment of recurrent anterior shoulder dislocation by the modified Bristow-Helfet procedure. S Afr Med J 65(9):325–330
41. Schroder DT, Provencher MT, Mologne TS, Muldoon MP, Cox JS (2006) The modified Bristow procedure for anterior shoulder instability: 26-year outcomes in Naval Academy midshipmen. Am J Sports Med 34(5):778–786

42. Lafosse L, Boyle S (2010) Arthroscopic Latarjet procedure. J Shoulder Elbow Surg 19(2 Suppl):2–12
43. Lafosse L, Boyle S, Gutierrez-Aramberri M, Shah A, Meller R (2010) Arthroscopic latarjet procedure. Orthop Clin North Am 41(3):393–405
44. Lafosse L, Lejeune E, Bouchard A, Kakuda C, Gobezie R, Kochhar T (2007) The arthroscopic Latarjet procedure for the treatment of anterior shoulder instability. Arthroscopy 23(11):1242 e1241–1245
45. Haaker RG, Eickhoff U, Klammer HL (1993) Intraarticular autogenous bone grafting in recurrent shoulder dislocations. Mil Med 158(3):164–169
46. Provencher MT, LeClere LE, Ghodadra N, Solomon DJ (2010) Postsurgical glenohumeral anchor arthropathy treated with a fresh distal tibia allograft to the glenoid and a fresh allograft to the humeral head. J Shoulder Elbow Surg 19(6):e6–11

Hill-Sachs Remplissage

7

Justin E. M. LeBlanc, Marie-Eve LeBel, Darren S. Drosdowech, Kenneth J. Faber and George S. Athwal

7.1 Introduction

Flower (1861) and Broca (1890) described a posterior superior humeral head defect that occurred secondarily after a glenohumeral joint dislocation [1, 2]. Hill and Sachs (1940) described this same entity as an impression fracture, seen on an anterior-posterior radiograph [3]. This impression fracture, which now bears their names, occurs in 57–70 % of first time anterior shoulder dislocations, and 94–100 % of recurrent dislocations [4–8]. Sizeable Hill-Sachs defects will decrease the rotational arc length of the humeral head on the glenoid, and have been associated with failed Bankart repairs due to engagement of the defect on the anterior rim of glenoid [5, 9–18].

A variety of methods can be utilized for treating patients with substantial Hill-Sachs defects including: retrograde defect elevation or humeroplasty, autograft or allograft reconstruction, proximal humeral rotational osteotomy, coracoid transfer to the glenoid, partial or complete arthroplasty, synthetic scaffolds, or filling of the defect with soft tissue [19]. The best treatment has not been defined in the current literature since some of these procedures address the defect directly, while others manipulate the articular arc length to prevent engagement of the defect on the glenoid rim. Connolly (1972) first described an open transfer of the infraspinatus tendon with a portion of the greater tuberosity into the posterior superior defect with satisfactory results in 14/15 patients [20]. An arthroscopic version of this procedure was developed and described as a remplissage, meaning "filling" in French [21, 22]. Remplissage is a non-anatomic technique that renders the defect extra-articular to prevent instability, using an arthroscopic posterior capsulodesis

J. E. M. LeBlanc · M.-E. LeBel · D. S. Drosdowech · K. J. Faber · G. S. Athwal (✉)
Shoulder Service, Hand and Upper Limb Centre (HULC), St Joseph's Health Care,
University of Western Ontario, 268 Grosvenor Street,
London, ON N6A 4L6, Canada
e-mail: gathwal@uwo.ca

S. F. Brockmeier et al. (eds.), *Surgery of Shoulder Instability*,
DOI: 10.1007/978-3-642-38100-3_7, © ISAKOS 2013

and infraspinatus tenodesis into the Hill-Sachs defect, performed in conjunction with a Bankart repair. The advantages of remplissage over other techniques are that it is an all arthroscopic solution that can be performed at the same time as a Bankart repair and uses local tissue without the need for foreign graft material.

7.2   Indications

Recurrence of anterior instability after isolated arthroscopic Bankart repair is higher in the presence of humeral bone loss [5, 11, 14]. Even with this known association, the critical size and orientation of the Hill-Sachs defect remains unknown and controversial. While most authors agree that Hill-Sachs defects less than 20 % can be treated non-operatively and those over 40 % should be treated operatively, it is those between 20 and 40 % that remain controversial, as they may be significant depending on their orientation, width and depth [23, 24]. Biomechanical studies have demonstrated that isolated Bankart repairs with a 15 % Hill-Sachs defect will not dislocate, while those with 30 and 45 % Hill-Sachs defect will dislocate prior to but not after remplissage [25–28]. Sekiya (2012) found that an isolated 25 % Hill-Sachs defect without anterior capsulolabral injury was stable, suggesting if the anterior capsulolabral injury heals, a 25 % Hill-Sachs defect may not be the critical size [29]. Recent review articles have suggested that remplissage be performed in patients with >25 % Hill-Sachs defect and glenoid loss less than 20–25 % [23, 30].

The orientation of the Hill-Sachs defect is important and determines the position of potential engagement [11]. Engagement has been used as an indication for surgery by multiple clinical studies [31–37] and is thought to be associated with up to a 100 % recurrence rate after isolated arthroscopic Bankart repair [9, 11]. The orientation, or Hill-Sachs angle, has been described as the angle between the longitudinal axis of the humerus and the deepest axis of the defect, which is more horizontal than non-engaging (25.6° vs. 13.8°) [38]. Yamamoto (2007) introduced the glenoid track concept [39]. It was felt that the orientation and width of the Hill-Sachs defect was of greater importance than depth and length. As the arm is normally elevated and externally rotated, the contact position between the glenoid and humeral head shifts from inferomedial to superolateral creating a "track". If the edge of the defect extends medial to the gleno-humeral contact area (track) in external rotation, the Hill-Sachs will likely engage with the glenoid rim. The track is normally 84 % of the glenoid length, and begins at the rotator cuff insertion on the greater tuberosity.

In summary, the critical width and angular orientation of a significant Hill-Sachs defect remains unknown. The above studies suggest some indications for remplissage: Hill-Sachs defect >25 % in width, glenoid bone loss <20 %, a more horizontal orientation/Hill-Sachs angle or engagement demonstrated during dynamic arthroscopic evaluation and a Hill-Sachs defect ending medial to the glenoid tract.

7.3   Evaluation

7.3.1   History and Physical Examination

The patient should be asked on the ease and frequency of dislocation/subluxations especially with activities of daily living and sleep, in addition to past traumatic events. Prior surgical interventions should also be elicited as bony instability is a common cause of failure [11, 40]. The physical exam should begin with routine inspection, comparative active and passive range of motion (ROM), strength, neurovascular exam, and an assessment of hyper-laxity. The regular instability special tests should be performed. A test that may be useful for bone loss, but requires further study, is the bony apprehension test [41]. In contrast to the traditional apprehension maneuver, this test demonstrates apprehension when performed at 45 ° of abduction and external rotation. This finding is supported by Kaar (2010) who found that larger Hill-Sachs defects where unstable at lesser degrees of motion than smaller defects [27].

7.3.2   Diagnostic Imaging

All instability cases should be evaluated for glenoid and humeral head bone loss with a standard shoulder radiographic series: AP glenoid (Grashey), axillary and trans-scapular Y lateral views. Additional views, such as the apical oblique (Garth) view provide a coronal profile of the gleno-humeral joint, with the ability to detect Hill-Sachs defect the posterosuperior head. Other useful views for evaluating Hill-Sachs defect are internal and external AP and Stryker notch views.

Cross sectional imaging is required to better evaluate bone loss. The Hill-Sachs defect should not be confused with the normal "bare area", which is a normal sulcus between the insertion of the posterior capsule and the edge of the articular cartilage along the humeral neck. Saito (2009) reported that the normal bare area will always begin 19 mm inferior to the top of the humeral head, whereas the Hill-Sachs defect will start anywhere from 0 to 24 mm below the humeral head [42]. Therefore, any defect between capsule and articular cartilage from 0 to 19 mm below humeral head is defined as a Hill-Sachs defect, below this mark being more difficult to distinguish between the two.

Computed tomography (CT) is the best choice for evaluating bone defects (Fig. 7.1a). It has been used to quantify bone loss (%) by dividing the defect arc with the humeral head arc [43]. The inter-observer correlation is 0.88–0.96 and 0.72–0.98 for depth and width respectively, with width often being underestimated and sagittal and axial cuts having lower errors versus coronal views for both depth and width [38, 44]. Magnetic resonance imaging (MRI) for the detection of Hill-Sachs defect demonstrates high sensitivity (0.96) and specificity (0.91), and high correlations ($\kappa = 0$), with moderate correlations to determine sizes greater or less than 1 cm ($\kappa = 0.44$) [45, 46]. The added benefit of MRI/MRA is the visualization of other soft tissue injuries. To the best of our knowledge, the use of MRI to determine Hill-Sachs

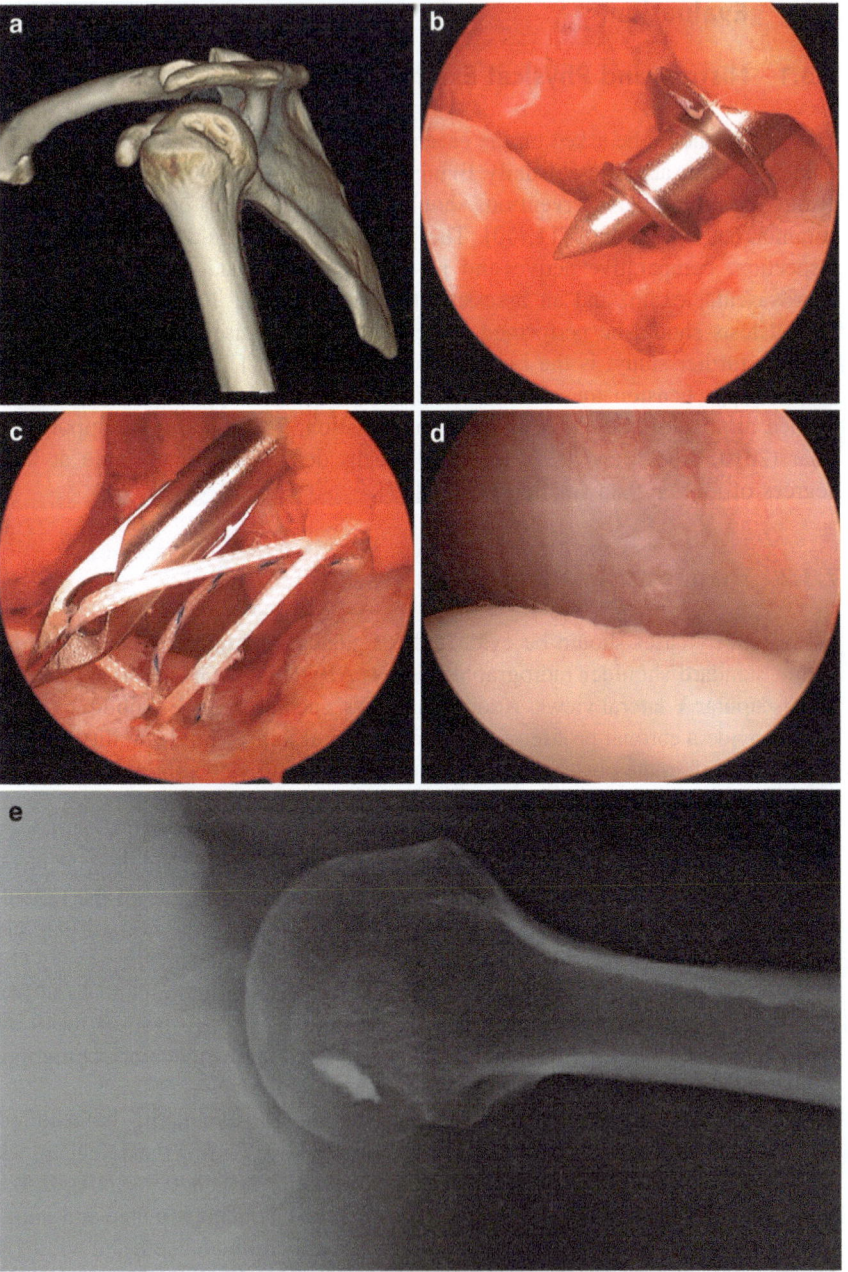

Fig. 7.1 A Hill-Sachs defect on a three dimensional CT reconstruction (**a**). Intra-operatively with the camera through the anterior portal, the prepared Hill-Sachs defect is visualized as is placement of a metallic anchor percutaneously through the posterior capsule and infraspinatus tendon (**b**). A penetrating instrument is used to create mattress sutures (**c**). Once the sutures are passes they are tied which results in "filling" of the Hill-Sachs defect (**d**). A post-operative axillary radiograph demonstrates two metallic anchors placed into the Hill-Sachs defect (**e**)

defect size and to predict engagement has not been evaluated. Ultrasound has also been described for detecting Hill-Sachs defects and has high reported sensitivity (0.96) and specificity (1.00). Ultrasound, however, cannot determine size or orientation [47] of the defect and the authors of this review have no experience with it.

7.4 Author's Recommended Technique

7.4.1 Goal

The goal of this surgery is filling of the abraded Hill-Sachs defect with the posterior capsule and infraspinatus tendon using suture anchors. Ideally this converts the defect into an extra-articular defect, preventing engagement and further dislocation (Fig. 7.1).

7.4.2 Set-Up

It is the authors' preference to position patients in the beach chair position. An exam under general anesthetic is gently performed for instability and engagement. The same portals for anterior instability surgery (Bankart repair) are used in this technique: a standard posterior portal, an anterior portal (within rotator interval, just above lateral half of subscapularis); and an anterosuperolateral portal (placed just inferior to the margin of the acromion, immediately anterior to the biceps tendon) are used.

7.4.3 Arthroscopy

A standard diagnostic arthroscopy is conducted. Bone loss of the glenoid and Hill-Sachs defects are evaluated. Dynamic engagement of the Hill-Sachs defect with the anterior edge of the glenoid is examined in various positions of abduction and external rotation. Engagement is evaluated more as a function of glenohumeral rotation in abduction-external rotation, rather than forced anterior humeral head translation. Begin with evaluation and preparation of the anterior labrum and glenoid. Prepare the Bankart lesion by passing sutures and placing anchors, but do not finish/tie until after the remplissage procedure is completed.

7.4.4 Remplissage Procedure

The arthroscope is positioned through the anterior portal. The humeral head can be translated anteriorly and externally rotated to improve visualization of the Hill-Sachs defect, as required. The standard posterior portal or an accessory posterolateral portal can be used to gently debride the Hill-Sachs defect with a curette, burr or shaver. The posterior capsule is also gently abraded. Typically, two anchors are placed into the defect (Fig. 7.1b). These anchors can be placed percutaneously or through the accessory posterolateral cannula. Prior to placement of the anchors, the posterior subdeltoid place is cleared of bursa to allow visualization during suture tying. A penetrating grasper is used percutaneously to penetrate the infraspinatus tendon and the posterior joint capsule to grasp a suture from the anchor to create mattress stitches (Figs. 7.1c and 7.2a). Care is taken to pass sutures through the adjacent joint capsule, not too medially as this may restrict range of motion [48]. Once all of the sutures are passed, the camera is placed in the subacromial space and the sutures are tied in the posterior subdeltoid space (Figs. 7.1d and 7.2b). During tying, the shoulder is reduced and the arm is placed in neutral rotation.

Once the remplissage is secured, the camera is returned to the gleno-humeral joint. The remplissage is evaluated and the Bankart repair is completed.

7.4.5 Post-operative

Patients are treated similarly to arthroscopic instability repairs with hand, wrist and elbow exercises started immediately. Patients are typically placed in a sling for 4–6 weeks. Pendulum exercises begin at 2–4 weeks, AAROM at 4–6 weeks. Abduction and external rotation beyond neutral are avoided until 6 weeks. Return to sports around 4–6 months.

7.4.6 Other Options

7.4.6.1 Lateral Decubitus Versus Beach Chair

Purchase (2008) suggests lateral decubitus with bed tilted posterior 30°, shoulder in 30° abduction and 15° forward flexion with 15 lbs of traction [21]. The remplissage should be performed in the position you are most comfortable performing arthroscopic anterior stabilization.

7.4.6.2 Position of Posterior Portal

A recent biomechanical study evaluated three different placements of anchors: placed in the defect valley (as originally described by Purchase [21]), in the humeral head rim (as described by Koo [33]), and in the valley with sutures placed medial [48]. Placement of sutures medially resulted in significantly greater stiffness and reduced internal-external ROM [48]. We suggest placing the anchor into the defect valley and ensuring sutures are passed thru the lateral tendon, immediately adjacent to the Hill-Sachs defect.

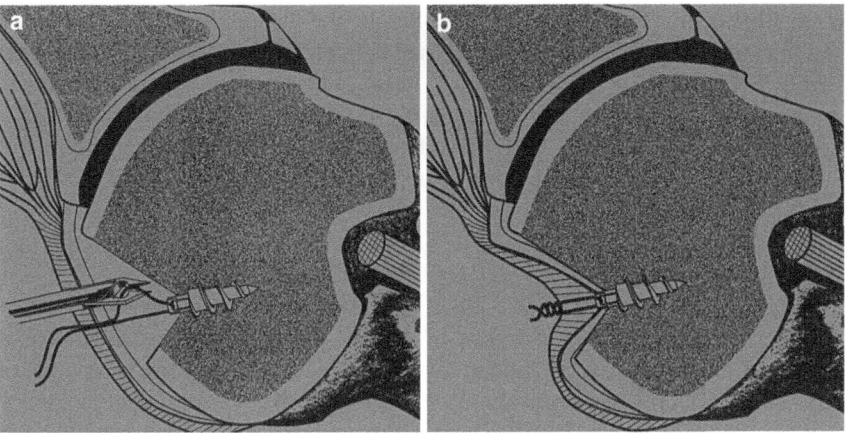

Fig. 7.2 A penetrating grasper is used to pass suture limbs inferior and superior to the anchor into the subdeltoid space (**a**). The limbs are then tied in the posterior subdeltoid space, creating a mattress suture through the posterior capsule and infraspinatus tendon (**b**)

7.4.6.3 Suture Technique

Purchase suggested a mattress suture technique [21]. Koo et al. introduced the double pulley technique as previously described in double row rotator cuff repair [33, 49]. This method is thought to provide a larger footprint of fixation and visualization of the knots over the infraspinatus tendon. At this time, there are no studies that confirm the amount of healing and footprint coverage required to restore stability. A recent MRI study demonstrated that stability is restored even when <0 % of the tendon has healed within the defect following remplissage [31].

7.5   Outcomes/Evidence

Our peer-reviewed literature search found nine English language clinical studies evaluating remplissage, one level II study, one level III, and seven level IV studies, all with short-term follow-up. Two studies compared a cohort of remplissage and Bankart repair alone procedures, and found no significant differences in postoperative range of motion or outcome scores [50], but a significantly higher dislocation rate in Bankart repair alone [51]. All studies have demonstrated an overall good outcome with low complication rates.

7.5.1   Recurrent Instability

Recurrent instability is defined as having subsequent dislocations, subluxations or positive apprehension tests after a repair. The recurrence rate ranges from 0 to 20 %, with an average of 6.6 % (14/212) [21, 31, 32, 34, 35, 37, 50–52]. Boileau et al. (2012) used minimal to no bone loss of the glenoid as their indication for remplissage and obtained lower recurrence rates of 2.1 % [31], compared to others using less than 25 % glenoid loss as their indications. Of these 14 recorded recurrences, 4 (28.6 %) were traumatic, 4 (28.6 %) were atraumatic with 3 spontaneous reductions, 3 (21.4 %) suffered subluxations, 2 (14.3 %) were from seizures, and 1 (7.1 %) had a positive apprehension test.

7.5.2 Range of Motion

Clinically, an average of 1.9–9° loss of external rotation and a loss of two spinal levels for internal rotation, without any patient dissatisfaction has been observed [31, 34, 37, 50]. This is comparable to the mean loss of 5.4° of external rotation for isolated Bankart repairs [18]. Deutsch (2008), however, reported a patient who experienced substantial loss of external rotation after a remplissage procedure [53]. This particular patient was treated with revision surgery.

7.5.3 Outcome Scores

Many different outcome scores are utilized in the remplissage outcome studies. The Western Ontario Shoulder Instability Index (WOSI) has been described as the most rigorously designed and evaluated, being both reliable and validated for instability [54]. All outcome scores demonstrated significant improvement from pre-operatively, with a post-operative average WOSI score of 72–74 % [34, 35], ASES 92–96 % [35, 37], and Rowe 80–91 % [31, 37].

7.5.4 Return to Work and Sport

A return to sporting activities and work are important outcome measures for young patients with instability. Return to sport is approximately 90 %, with 68–80 % returning to the same level as pre-injury [31, 37, 51]. Most (80–100 %) of professional athletes return to their same level [31, 52], and up to 100 % of patients return to their work [52].

7.5.5 Healing

At least partial healing of the remplissage is shown in 100 % of patients, with >74 % of patients demonstrating healing of >75 % of the footprint by MRI or CT arthrogram [31, 34, 37, 50, 51]. It is difficult to calculate the exact percentage of healing using MRI due to artifact from the anchors [50], but by adding contrast to a CT, the assessment of healing is improved [31]. At this time we are unsure what percentage of healing is required, as even patients with <50 % healing at 6 months demonstrate no recurrence [31]. Secondary findings in these MRIs demonstrated up to 44 % of patients having partial infraspinatus tears or tendinopathy, and 0–25 % fatty infiltration of their infraspinatus [34].

7.5.6   Complications

Recurrence and posterior shoulder pain are the most frequent complications observed following remplissage. Posterior shoulder pain with forceful movements or when the arm was fatigued are noted in 2–33 % of patients [31, 50]. This is felt to be secondary to partial healing or more likely due to impingement between the posterior labrum with the new location of the footprint of the posterior cuff [50]. A recent biomechanical study reported data consistent with this clinical finding, with the soft tissue bumper being abutted against the glenoid in lesser degrees of extension and external rotation [26].

7.5.7   Biomechanics

Biomechanical studies have evaluated stability of the glenohumeral joint, joint stiffness and internal–external rotational range of motion (IE-ROM) changes after the remplissage procedure. Bankart repair alone failed to prevent dislocations with Hill-Sachs defects of 30 and 45 %, while those with 15 % were stable [25, 26]. Remplissage prevented dislocation in all 3 sizes of defects [25, 26]. Remplissage significantly reduced IE-ROM in adduction for 15 and 30 % Hill-Sachs defect compared to intact state and Bankart repair alone [25, 26]. Stiffness was significantly increased for 15 % Hill-Sachs defect repaired with remplissage compared to Bankart repair alone, while remplissage for 30 and 45 % defects restored joint to near normal, with no significant difference to Bankart repair alone [25, 26].

7.6   Summary

Arthroscopic remplissage with anterior capsulolabral (Bankart) repair for moderate to large engaging Hill-Sachs defects with minimal glenoid bone loss has predictable healing, good quality of life outcome scores, and most patients return to sport at the same level. While biomechanical and clinical studies demonstrate a loss in external rotation, this loss of rotation may not be clinically important. We suggest remplissage as a procedure for patients with engaging Hill-Sachs defects with minimal glenoid bone loss (<20 %). Longer-term prospective and comparative studies are still needed to fully evaluate remplissage outcomes, specifically evaluating how stiffness and loss of range of motion affect work and sports.

References

1. Broca A, Hartmann H (1890) Contribution a l'etude des luxations de l'epaule (Luxations anciennes, luxations recidivantes). Bulletins de la Societe Anatomique de Paris 5
2. Flower WH (1861) On the pathological changes produced in the shoulder-joint by traumatic dislocation: as derived from an examination of all the specimens illustrating this injury in the museums of London
3. Hill HA, Sachs MD (1940) The grooved defect of the humeral head: a frequently unrecognized complication of dislocations of the shoulder joint. Radiology 35(6):690–700
4. Antonio GE, Griffith JF, Yu AB, Yung PSH, Chan KM, Ahuja AT (2007) First-time shoulder dislocation: high prevalence of labral injury and age-related differences revealed by MR arthrography. J Magn Reson Imaging 26(4):983–991
5. Boileau P, Villalba M, Hery JY, Balg F, Ahrens P, Neyton L (2006) Risk factors for recurrence of shoulder instability after arthroscopic Bankart repair. J Bone Joint Surg 88(8):1755–1763
6. Bushnell BD, Creighton RA, Herring MM (2008) Bony instability of the shoulder. Arthrosc: J Arthrosc & Relat Surg 24(9):1061–1073
7. Kim DS, Yoon YS, Yi CH (2010) Prevalence comparison of accompanying lesions between primary and recurrent anterior dislocation in the shoulder. Am J Sports Med 38(10):2071–2076
8. Yiannakopoulos CK, Mataragas E, Antonogiannakis E (2007) A comparison of the spectrum of intra-articular lesions in acute and chronic anterior shoulder instability. Arthrosc: J Arthrosc & Relat Surg 23(9):985–990
9. Ahmed I, Ashton F, Robinson CM (2012) Arthroscopic Bankart repair and capsular shift for recurrent anterior shoulder instability functional outcomes and identification of risk factors for recurrence. J Bone Joint Surg 94(14):1308–1315
10. Burkhart SS, Danaceau SM (2000) Articular arc length mismatch as a cause of failed Bankart repair. Arthrosc: J Arthrosc & Relat Surg 16(7):740–744
11. Burkhart SS, De Beer JF (2000) Traumatic glenohumeral bone defects and their relationship to failure of arthroscopic Bankart repairs. Arthrosc: J Arthrosc & Relat Surg 16(7):677–694
12. Cetik O, Uslu M, Ozsar BK (2007) The relationship between Hill-Sachs lesion and recurrent anterior shoulder dislocation. Acta Orthop Belg 73(2):175
13. Flinkkila T, Hyvonen P, Ohtonen P, Leppilahti J (2010) Arthroscopic Bankart repair: results and risk factors of recurrence of instability. Knee Surg Sports Traumatol Arthrosc 18(12):1752–1758
14. Kralinger FS, Golser K, Wischatta R, Wambacher M, Sperner G (2002) Predicting recurrence after primary anterior shoulder dislocation. Am J Sports Med 30(1):116–120
15. Lynch JR, Clinton JM, Dewing CB, Warme WJ, Matsen FA III (2009) Treatment of osseous defects associated with anterior shoulder instability. J Shoulder Elbow Surg 18(2):317–328
16. Palmer I, Widen A (1948) The bone block method for recurrent dislocation of the shoulder joint. J Bone Joint Surg Br 30(1):53
17. Rowe C, Zarins B, Ciullo J (1984) Recurrent anterior dislocation of the shoulder after surgical repair. Apparent causes of failure and treatment. J Bone Joint Surg Am 66(2):159–168
18. Voos JE, Livermore RW, Feeley BT, Altchek DW, Williams RJ, Warren RF et al (2010) Prospective evaluation of arthroscopic Bankart repairs for anterior instability. Am J Sports Med 38(2):302–307
19. Armitage MS, Faber KJ, Drosdowech DS, Litchfield RB, Athwal GS (2010) Humeral head bone defects: remplissage, allograft, and arthroplasty. Orthop Clin North Am 41(3):417–425. doi:10.1016/j.ocl.2010.03.004
20. Connolly J (1972) Humeral head defects associated with shoulder dislocation. J Am Acad Orthop Surg Instr Course Lectures 11:42–54

21. Purchase RJ, Wolf EM, Hobgood ER, Pollock ME, Smalley CC (2008) Hill-Sachs remplissage: an arthroscopic solution for the engaging Hill-Sachs lesion. Arthrosc: J Arthrosc & Relat Surg 24(6):723–726
22. Wolf EM, Pollack ME (2004) Hill-Sachs remplissage: an arthroscopic solution for the engaging Hill-Sachs lesion (SS-32). Arthrosc: J Arthrosc & Relat Surg 20:e14–e15
23. Bollier MJ, Arciero R (2010) Management of glenoid and humeral bone loss. Sports Med Arthrosc Rev 18(3):140–148
24. Skendzel JG, Sekiya JK (2012) Diagnosis and management of humeral head bone loss in shoulder instability. Am J Sports Med 40(11):2633–2644. doi:10.1177/0363546512437314
25. Elkinson I, Giles JW, Faber KJ, Boons HW, Ferreira LM, Johnson JA et al (2012) The effect of the remplissage procedure on shoulder stability and range of motion. J Bone Joint Surg Am 94:1003–1012
26. Giles JW, Elkinson I, Ferreira LM, Faber KJ, Boons H, Litchfield R et al (2011) Moderate to large engaging Hill-Sachs defects: an in vitro biomechanical comparison of the remplissage procedure, allograft humeral head reconstruction, and partial resurfacing arthroplasty. J Shoulder Elbow Surg 21(9):1142–1151. doi:10.1016/j.jse.2011.07.017
27. Kaar SG, Fening SD, Jones MH, Colbrunn RW, Miniaci A (2010) Effect of humeral head defect size on glenohumeral stability: a cadaveric study of simulated Hill-Sachs defects. Am J Sports Med 38(3):594–599
28. Sekiya JK, Wickwire AC, Stehle JH, Debski RE (2009) Hill-Sachs defects and repair using osteoarticular allograft transplantation biomechanical analysis using a joint compression model. Am J Sports Med 37(12):2459–2466
29. Sekiya JK, Jolly J, Debski RE (2012) The effect of a Hill-Sachs defect on glenohumeral translations, in situ capsular forces, and bony contact forces. Am J Sports Med 40(2):388–394
30. Provencher M, Bhatia S, Ghodadra N, Grumet R, Bach B Jr, Dewing C et al (2010) Recurrent shoulder instability: current concepts for evaluation and management of glenoid bone loss. J Bone Joint Surg Am 92(Suppl 2):133–151. doi:10.2106/JBJS.J.00906
31. Boileau P, O'Shea K, Vargas P, Pinedo M, Old J, Zumstein M (2012) Anatomical and functional results after arthroscopic Hill-Sachs remplissage. J Bone Joint Surg 94(7):618–626
32. Gracitelli MEC, Helito CP, Malavolta EA, Neto AAF, Benegas E, de Santis-Prada F et al (2011) Results from filling "remplissage" arthroscopic technique for recurrent anterior shoulder dislocation. Rev Bras Ortop 46(6):684–690
33. Koo SS, Burkhart SS, Ochoa E (2009) Arthroscopic double-pulley remplissage technique for engaging Hill-Sachs lesions in anterior shoulder instability repairs. Arthrosc: J Arthrosc & Relat Surg 25(11):1343–1348
34. Park MJ, Garcia G, Malhotra A, Major N, Tjoumakaris FP, Kelly JD (2012) The evaluation of arthroscopic remplissage by high-resolution magnetic resonance imaging. Am J Sports Med 40(10):2331–2336. doi:10.1177/0363546512456974
35. Park MJ, Tjoumakaris FP, Garcia G, Patel A, Kelly JD (2011) Arthroscopic remplissage with Bankart repair for the treatment of glenohumeral instability with Hill-Sachs defects. Arthrosc: J Arthrosc & Relat Surg 27(9):1187–1194
36. Toro F, Melean P, Moraga C, Ruiz F, Gonzalez F, Vaisman A (2008) Remplissage: infraspinatus tenodesis and posterior capsulodesis for the treatment of Hill-Sachs lesions: an all intraarticular technique. Tech Shoulder Elbow Surg 9(4):188–192
37. Zhu YM, Lu Y, Zhang J, Shen JW, Jiang CY (2011) Arthroscopic Bankart repair combined with remplissage technique for the treatment of anterior shoulder instability with engaging Hill-Sachs lesion: a report of 49 cases with a minimum 2-year follow-up. Am J Sports Med 39(8):1640–1647
38. Cho SH, Cho NS, Rhee YG (2011) Preoperative analysis of the Hill-Sachs lesion in anterior shoulder instability how to predict engagement of the lesion. Am J Sports Med 39(11):2389–2395

39. Yamamoto N, Itoi E, Abe H, Minagawa H, Seki N, Shimada Y et al (2007) Contact between the glenoid and the humeral head in abduction, external rotation, and horizontal extension: a new concept of glenoid track. J Shoulder Elbow Surg 16(5):649–656
40. Tauber M, Resch H, Forstner R, Raffl M, Schauer J (2004) Reasons for failure after surgical repair of anterior shoulder instability. J Shoulder Elbow Surg 13(3):279–285
41. Bushnell BD, Creighton RA, Herring MM (2008) The bony apprehension test for instability of the shoulder: a prospective pilot analysis. Arthrosc: J Arthrosc & Relat Surg 24(9):974–982
42. Saito H, Itoi E, Minagawa H, Yamamoto N, Tuoheti Y, Seki N (2009) Location of the Hill-Sachs lesion in shoulders with recurrent anterior dislocation. Arch Orthop Trauma Surg 129(10):1327–1334
43. Montgomery WH Jr, Wahl M, Hettrich C, Itoi E, Lippitt SB, Matsen FA III (2005) Anteroinferior bone-grafting can restore stability in osseous glenoid defects. J Bone Joint Surg 87(9):1972–1977
44. Kodali P, Jones MH, Polster J, Miniaci A, Fening SD (2011) Accuracy of measurement of Hill-Sachs lesions with computed tomography. J Shoulder Elbow Surg 20(8):1328–1334
45. Hayes ML, Collins MS, Morgan JA, Wenger DE, Dahm DL (2010) Efficacy of diagnostic magnetic resonance imaging for articular cartilage lesions of the glenohumeral joint in patients with instability. Skeletal Radiol 39(12):1199–1204
46. Kirkley A, Litchfield R, Thain L, Spouge A (2003) Agreement between magnetic resonance imaging and arthroscopic evaluation of the shoulder joint in primary anterior dislocation of the shoulder. Clin J Sport Med 13(3):148–151
47. Cicak N, Bilic R, Delimar D (1998) Hill-Sachs lesion in recurrent shoulder dislocation: sonographic detection. J Ultrasound Med 17(9):557–560
48. Elkinson I, Giles JW, Boons HW, Faber KJ, Ferreira LM, Johnson JA et al (2012) The shoulder remplissage procedure for Hill-Sachs defects: does technique matter? J Shoulder Elbow Surg (Epub ahead of print). doi:10.1016/j.jse.2012.08.015
49. Arrigoni P, Brady PC, Burkhart SS (2007) The double-pulley technique for double-row rotator cuff repair. Arthrosc: J Arthrosc & Relat Surg 23(6):675.e1–675.e4
50. Nourissat G, Kilinc AS, Werther JR, Doursounian L (2011) A prospective, comparative, radiological, and clinical study of the influence of the remplissage procedure on shoulder range of motion after stabilization by arthroscopic Bankart repair. Am J Sports Med 39(10):2147–2152
51. Franceschi F, Papalia R, Rizzello G, Franceschetti E, Del Buono A, Panasci M et al (2012) Remplissage repair—new frontiers in the prevention of recurrent shoulder instability: a 2-year follow-up comparative study. Am J Sports Med 40(11):2462–2469. doi:10.1177/0363546512458572
52. Haviv B, Mayo L, Biggs D (2011) Outcomes of arthroscopic "remplissage": capsulotenodesis of the engaging large Hill-Sachs lesion. J Orthop Surg Res 6(1):29
53. Deutsch AA, Kroll DG (2008) Decreased range of motion following arthroscopic remplissage. Orthopedics 31(5):492
54. Plancher KD, Lipnick SL (2009) Analysis of evidence-based medicine for shoulder instability. Arthrosc: J Arthrosc & Relat Surg 25(8):897–908

Surgical Management of Posterior Shoulder Instability

8

Gernot Seppel, Sepp Braun and Andreas B. Imhoff

8.1 Introduction

Affecting only 2 % of the general population glenohumeral instability is a rare condition [1] According to the literature 2–10 % of all patients with shoulder instability present with posterior instability [2–11]. This condition is frequently found in young athletic patients, especially playing sports like football or rugby, climbing or weight lifting.

Posterior shoulder instability is sometimes difficult to diagnose and still management can be challenging due to the complexity of pathogenetic factors. Owing to the varying spectrum of clinical symptoms posterior instability of the shoulder can mimic various other pathologies like outlet impingement or lesions of the long head of the biceps tendon, or can be simply missed [12]. As symptoms in posterior instability are induced by an abnormal posterior translation of the humeral head relative to the glenoid rim, most patients complain about generalized and vague activity-related shoulder pain as well as reduction of activities including a loss of strength. Patients often report having difficulties in pushing heavy doors open [13].

In contrast to the thicker and more stable anterior glenohumeral joint capsule with its reinforcing ligamentous structures (SGHL, MGHL, IGHL), the posterior capsule is only supported by the posterior band of the inferior glenohumeral ligament (pIGHL), which is relatively thin and biomechanically less rugged [14]. Beside the bony anatomy, the capsulolabral structures are the most important static

G. Seppel · S. Braun
Department of Orthopaedic Sports Medicine, Technical University of Munich, Munich, Germany

A. B. Imhoff (✉)
Department of Orthopaedic Sports Medicine, Technical University Munich, Ismaninger Str. 22, 81675 Munich, Germany
e-mail: a.imhoff@lrz.tum.de

S. F. Brockmeier et al. (eds.), *Surgery of Shoulder Instability*,
DOI: 10.1007/978-3-642-38100-3_8, © ISAKOS 2013

stabilizers of the shoulder joint [15–17]. Injury or inherent abnormalities of these structures like an increased volume of the posteroinferior capsular pouch [18], dysplasia of the posterior chondrolabral rim [19] or bony glenoid retroversion [9] can result in instability. The primary dynamic stabilizer is the subscapularis muscle [17, 20]. This has to be taken into consideration during clinical examination as well as during diagnostic arthroscopy.

To understand the complexity of the diagnosis of "posterior shoulder instability" it is essential to meticulously analyze the pathology.

As the underlying pathogenesis indicates the treatment strategies, Lévigne et al. [21, 22] suggest the following classification:

- Primary posterior luxation.
- Chronic posterior instability without hyperlaxity.
- Chronic posterior instability with hyperlaxity (involuntary).
- Chronic posterior instability with hyperlaxity (voluntary).

The etiology of recurrent posterior shoulder instability includes repeated microtraumata, single traumatic events or atraumatic causes [23].

Repetitive microtraumata in a forward flexed and internally rotated position (e.g. swimming, rowing, bench press lifting etc.) is the most frequent cause of chronic posterior instability and can lead to injury of the posterior labrum [9] as well as to the pIGHL and the adjacent capsular structures [23, 24].

Traumatic posterior instability can typically be associated with a history of an acute injury like a posteriorly directed blow to the arm.

The rarest cause of posterior instability is general ligamentous laxity, which is not associated with any trauma. Patients usually suffer from progressive pain and sensation of instability in daily living that may have initially be present only in extensive activities or provocative positions like flexion, adduction and internal rotation [11]. Not rarely patients characterize an ability to "voluntarily" subluxate their glenohumeral joint posteriorly.

Millet et al. [25] describe two types of voluntary glenohumeral instability: voluntary positional and voluntary muscular.

Habitual or voluntary muscular instability indicates an underlying muscular imbalance or ligamentous laxity and is non position-dependent. As these patients do not present with the actual pathogenetic factors of recurrent posterior instability they typically do not qualify for surgical treatment [25].

In contrast to voluntary muscular instability, patients with voluntary positional instability can provoke subluxation in a forward flexed and internally rotated position. These candidates benefit from surgical treatment [26].

8.2   Indication

In general all patients with posterior instability should initially be treated non-operative. This should include physical therapy focusing on muscle strengthening and proprioception training programs [27, 28]. There are reports that both pain and instability can be reduced especially in patients with general ligamentous laxity and a history of repetitive microtrauma to the shoulder joint (atraumatic subluxators) [27–29]. For this group of patients rehabilitation can succeed in 70–89 % [27]. Patients with distinct traumatic events or posterior labral tears are less responsive to physical therapy and rehabilitation programs [8] with a success rate of only 16 % in case of post-traumatic recurrent subluxationsw [27].

Arthroscopic posterior stabilization is indicated in younger patients with isolated posterior instability suffering from persistent pain and instability and unsuccessful precedent comprehensive non-operative treatment [13, 28, 29]. Increased glenoid retroversion or bone loss needs to be ruled out.

Nevertheless, preoperative specific strengthening of the dynamic stabilizers of the scapula and the subscapularis muscle, the most important dynamic stabilizer of the posterior glenohumeral joint, is crucial for success of rehabilitation programs [9].

Within the group of multidirectional instability patients who have failed physical therapy and persistently suffer from posterior-inferior instability may benefit from a simple posterior capsular shift or plication.

Arthroscopic posterior stabilization is suggested for patients with isolated labral repair whereas open procedure should be favored in failed arthroscopic management or higher grades of posterior laxity in clinical exam [13]. Patients with poor capsular tissue or excessive glenoid retroversion require open surgery too.

The first patient cohorts undergoing open surgery for posterior instability in the 1980s and 1990s were reported with high recurrence rates, low patient satisfaction and delay or inability to return to sports [28–33]. High failure rates of 30–70 % are described for open procedures, possibly due to the extensive dissection and the inability to visualize all of the pathologic tissues [9] as well as the unique biomechanical properties of the posteroinferior capsule and labrum [11, 30]. In patients with significant bone loss or glenoid retroversion, open procedures like glenoid osteotomy [34], bone blocks [35] or in very limited special cases rotational osteotomy of the proximal humerus [4] can be indicated.

Due to less operative dissection and easier access to the posterior capsulolabral complex arthroscopic posterior shoulder stabilization is the treatment of choice in patients without substantial bone loss [9].

8.3   Diagnostics

A meticulous clinical exam of both shoulders is essential for diagnosing the correct etiology of a patient's complaints. The clinical findings should be re-evaluated under anesthesia in case of decision for surgical proceeding [36].

Regularly range of motion testing in patients with posterior instability is normal on both shoulders [28] and positive signs of apprehension are uncommon. By performing specific posteroinferior provocative translation testing maneuvers, posterior instability can be found and the grade and direction of instability can be determined with help of the Jerk test [37], the Kim test [38] and the load and shift test [39].

The Jerk test [37] is performed by axial posterior loading onto a 90° flexed, adducted and internally rotated arm. A positive test results in reproducing the instability sensation associated with pain as the subluxed humeral head relocates into the glenoid fossa [9].

Another sensitive test is the Kim test [38]. With the patient sitting the arm is brought to 90° of abduction and the examiner grasps the lateral proximal humerus to apply an axial loading force. With the examiners other hand the patient's elbow is held. The test is positive if the patients complaines about a sudden onset of pain when the arm is elevated to 45° with postero-inferiorly directed load to the upper arm.

Positive findings in both, the Jerk test and the Kim test, are up to 97 % sensitive for posterior instability [38].

For the load and shift test [39] the patient's arm is held at 20° forward flexion and is abducted. The test is performed in supine position with anterior and posterior loading to the humeral head. In a positive test pain or subluxation can be reproduced.

Imaging of the shoulder starts with radiographs. Standard series (AP view, axillary view, scapular Y view) often show normal findings, but they may be useful to appreciate the osseous anatomy of the glenoid and the humeral head.

Magnetic resonance imaging (MRI) and magnetic resonance arthrography (MRA) enable visualization of multiple capsulolabral components, the biceps anchor, the rotator cuff and the rotator interval that are essential for diagnosing posterior instability and planning operative treatment. Furthermore concomitant injuries to the capsular insertion on the humerus (pHAGL = posterior humeral avulsion of the glenohumeral ligament) can be detected reliably.

For assessing the osseous anatomy and pathologies like glenoid hypoplasia, glenoid retroversion or glenoid bone loss computed tomography is beneficial and important for operative planning.

8.4   Operative Technique

Before starting surgery a thorough examination of the shoulder under anesthesia should be performed. In order to assess any side-differences it is important to examine both shoulders. Beside range of motion, the grade of posterior instability should be confirmed under anesthesia.

8.4.1 Arthroscopic Surgical Technique

Indication for arthroscopic procedures include.

- chronic posterior instability without hyperlaxity,
- chronic posterior instability without bony posterior deficiency and
- posterior humeral avulsion of the glenohumeral ligaments (pHAGL).

Relative Contraindications are

- posterior instability due to glenoid dysplasia
- chronic posterior instability with hyperlaxity (voluntary)
- locked posterior dislocation
- major bony humeral defects (Malgaigne impressions with involvement of >25 % of the articulating surface).

For better distraction we prefer the lateral decubitus position with the patient's head facing towards the surgeon into the theater. Thereby the inferior and posterior quadrants of the shoulder get opened more effectively [40] and the complete glenohumeral joint can be approached (Fig. 8.1).

Via a 3-point traction sleeve the 50° abducted and 15° flexed arm gets pulled laterally and distally (Fig. 8.2).

After marking the anatomical landmarks the portals are established as shown above. The posterior standard portal, the anterosuperior portal and a posterolateral portal (Fig. 8.3).

A diagnostic arthroscopy starting from the posterior standard portal is done in every case. By evaluating the posterior labrum the need to perform a labral repair or a capsular shift can be assessed. Furthermore it allows the identification of concomitant pathologies, e.g. SLAP tears, biceps tendon lesions or chondral injuries.

Subsequently the anterosuperior portal is established just anterior to the acromioclavicular joint by localizing the correct position with a spinal needle and inserting a 8.25/7 mm threaded cannula. Via this portal and its 12-o'clock view the posterior labrum, the capsule and the posterior glenoid all the way down to the axillary pouch can be thoroughly visualized. Additionally a midglenoid portal just above the subscapularis tendon with a 6 mm cannula can be inserted for labral evaluation,preparation and suture management.

For posterior stabilization one additional posterior portal is mandatory because usually the posteroinferior aspect of the glenohumeral joint cannot be assessed sufficiently through the posterior standard viewing portal.

This deep posterolateral portal is placed in a 7-o'clock position 2–3 cm lateral to the posterior corner of the acromion and a working cannula with flaps (Gemini, Arthrex Inc, Naples, FL, USA) is inserted. To enable passage of instruments larger (7–8 mm) cannulas must be placed. The posterolateral portal provides excellent access [5] for inserting anchors biomechanically optimal at an angle of 135° to the glenoid plane. But one should be aware that there is a potential risk for injury of the posterior axillary nerve with this portal. To avoid this only a superficial skin

Fig. 8.1 Lateral position, patient's head towards surgeon

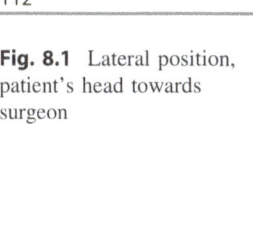

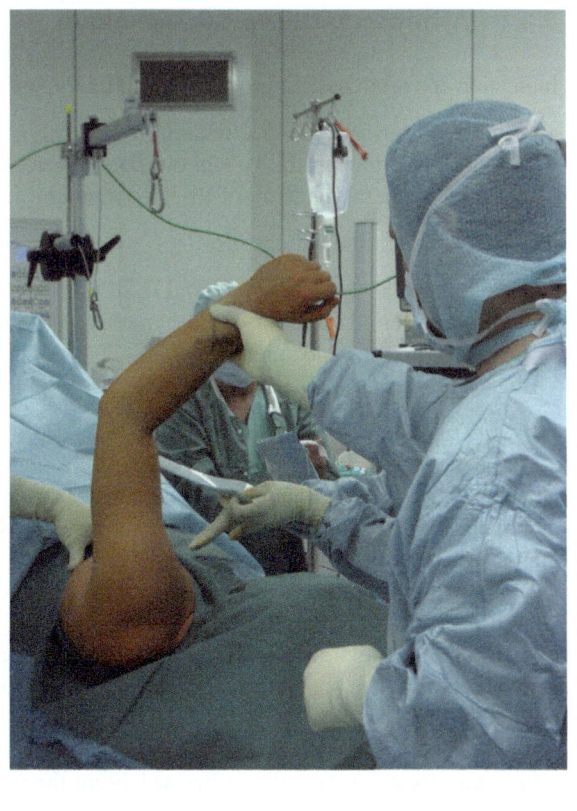

Fig. 8.2 Lateral decubitus: The arm is 50° abducted and 15° flexed

Fig. 8.3 Anatomical
landmarks (A = Acromion;
Cl = Clavicle;
Co = Coracoid; x = portals
(see also Fig. 8.4))

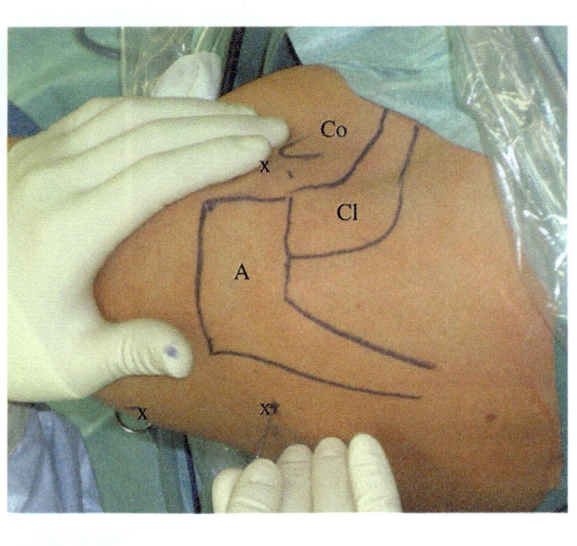

incision is performed and a blunt Wissinger rod is introduced into the joint as a guide for the cannula (Fig. 8.4).

The first step in performing a posterior labral tear is to extensively mobilize the posterior labrum (Fig. 8.5).

Using the 12 o'clock view with the arthroscope in the anterosuperior portal, the labrum can be carefully elevated off the surface of the glenoid neck with a Bankart knife introduced through the posterolateral portal (Fig. 8.6).

Fig. 8.4 Portal positioning:
anterior: anterosuperior
portal; posterior standard
portal; deep posterolateral
portal with a special cannula
(Gemini Cannula
incorporates a deployable
wing to keep the capsule
away and to prevent cannula
"fall-out" during insertion).
(Figure originally
from: "Imhoff, Feucht—Atlas
sportorthopädisch-
sporttraumatologische
Operationen", Springer, 2012)

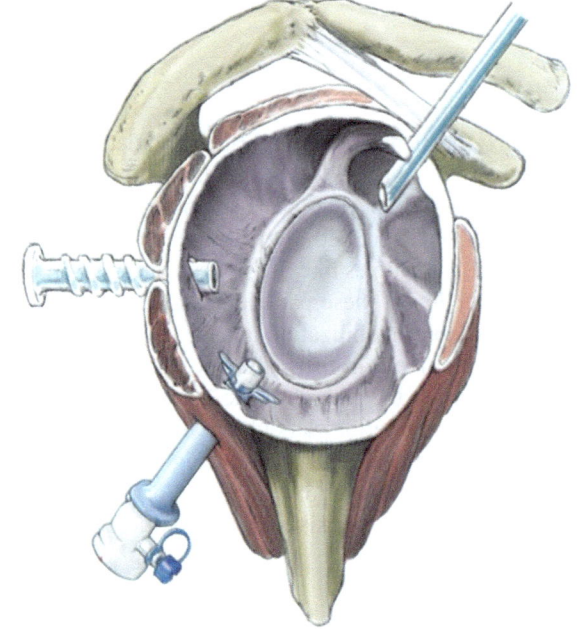

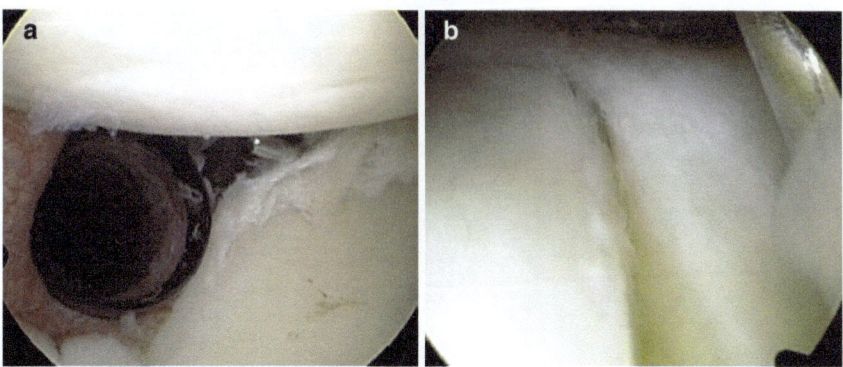

Fig. 8.5 View from the 12 o'clock view towards the two posterior portals and the posterior labrum

Fig. 8.6 Mobilization of the labrum and debridement of the glenoid rim

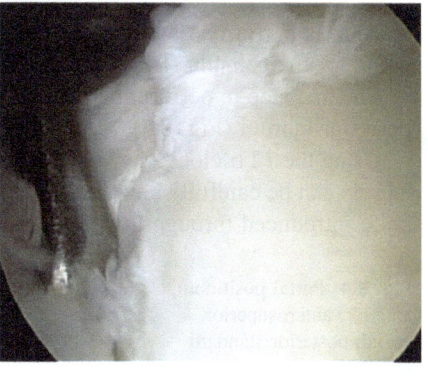

Next the glenoid rim is debrided and decorticated with a rasp to achieve a fresh bleeding bony surface. It is important to address the most inferior aspect of the glenohumeral joint first, because posterior shoulder volume and working space is progressively narrowed after each capsulolabral repair stitch. Subsequently concomitant pathologies like SLAP lesions can be addressed but some surgeons prefer reconstruction of these pathologies at the very beginning.

After labral mobilization anchor positions are identified and marked carefully either with an electrothermal device or an arthroscopic burr into the glenoid rim. Depending on the extend of the labral lesion we tend to use 2–4 anchors placed right on the posterior glenoid rim. Routinely we insert at least two anchors at 7-o'clock and one at 8.30-o'clock (Fig. 8.7).

For isolated posterior labral and/or capsular injuries this may be sufficient whereas in more extensive lesions additional anchors or capsular plications can be needed.

Fig. 8.7 Anchor positioning (Figure originally from: "Imhoff, Feucht—Atlas sportorthopädisch-sporttraumatologische Operationen", Springer, 2012)

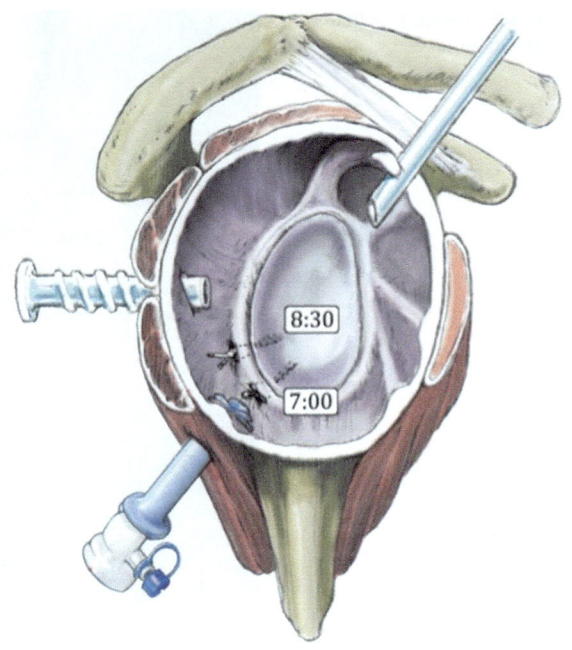

In patients with minor posterior capsular laxity a capsular plication can be done by piercing the joint capsule approximately 1 cm lateral to the labrum with a 45-degree curved (left 45-degree curved for left shoulders and vice versa) suture lasso passer (Arthrex Inc, Naples, FL, USA).

For labral repair and capsular shift the labrum gets penetrated with the same suture passer just inferior to the anchor with helps to pull the capsulolabral complex superiorly (Figs. 8.8 and 8.9).

After drilling the anchors are inserted through the accessory posterior portal as shown above. Typically we use bioabsorbable anchors. One limb of the suture is pulled through the portal with the lasso while the other limb gets pulled out by an arthroscopic retriever (Figs. 8.10 and 8.11).

The sliding knot is tied outside the joint and pulled down sitting posterior to the labral complex. These steps are repeated until the complete labrum is reattached (Figs. 8.12 and 8.13).

In patients with multidirectional instability a closure of the rotator cuff interval can be performed.

Capsular plication is performed to reduce the volume of a widened capsule and to strengthen the posterior soft tissue restraints of the joint. It is essential to avoid overtightening as this may result in significantly decreased range of motion, especially internal rotation. Determining the amount of capsular plication can be challenging. In general a 1 cm plication of the posteroinferior aspects of the capsule with 1–3 sutures is an adequate correction.

Fig. 8.8 Labral penetration
with suture lasso

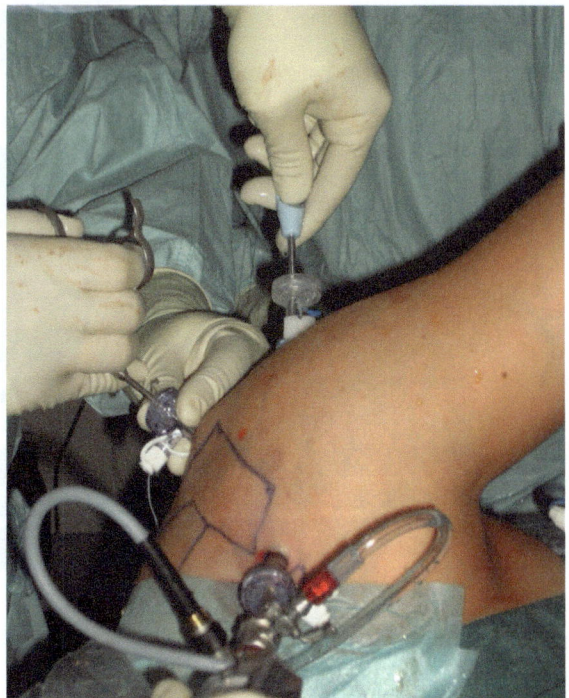

Fig. 8.9 Penetration of the
labrum and shuttling of the
sutures with a suture lasso

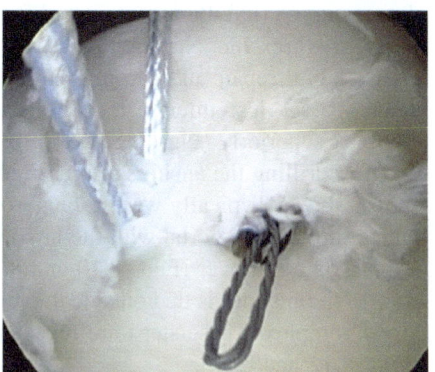

Although singular capsular plication is described as adequate therapeutic option in patients without a pathologic labrum [8] we routinely use anchor fixation for posterior stabilization in general.

In case of hyperlaxity, it is recommended to perform a plication of the anterior-inferior joint capsule aspect additionally to the posterior labral repair [41].

Although reducing the volume of the capsule is essential for a successful operative procedure t overtightening of the shoulder needs to be avoided [42, 43].

Fig. 8.10 Drilling at the
glenoid rim

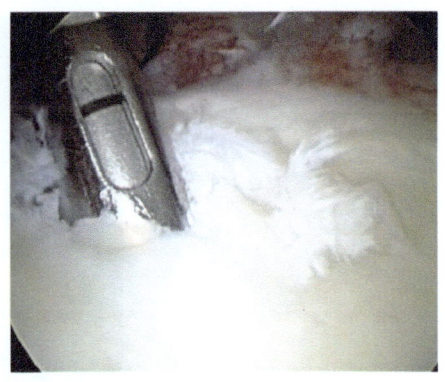

Fig. 8.11 Inserting the
anchor

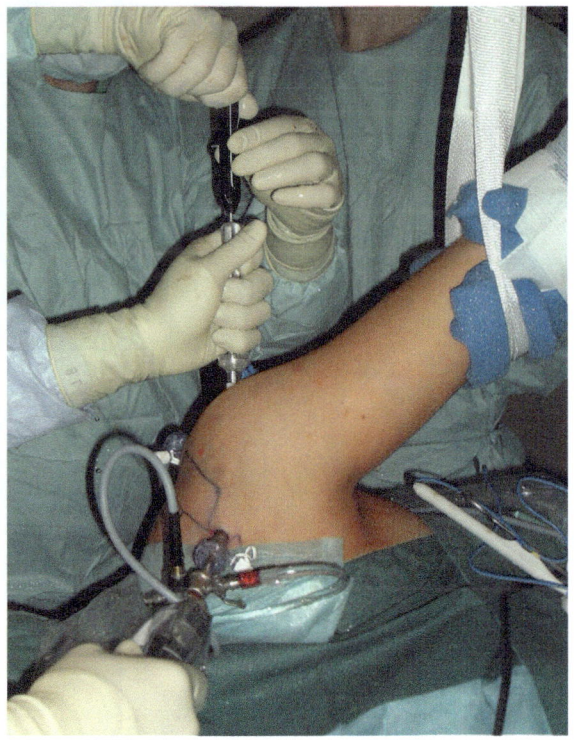

8.4.2   Open Surgical Technique

Open treatment options:

1. Open wedge osteotomy of the glenoid.
2. Posterior bone block procedure.

Fig. 8.12 Tying of the
sliding knot outside the
cannula

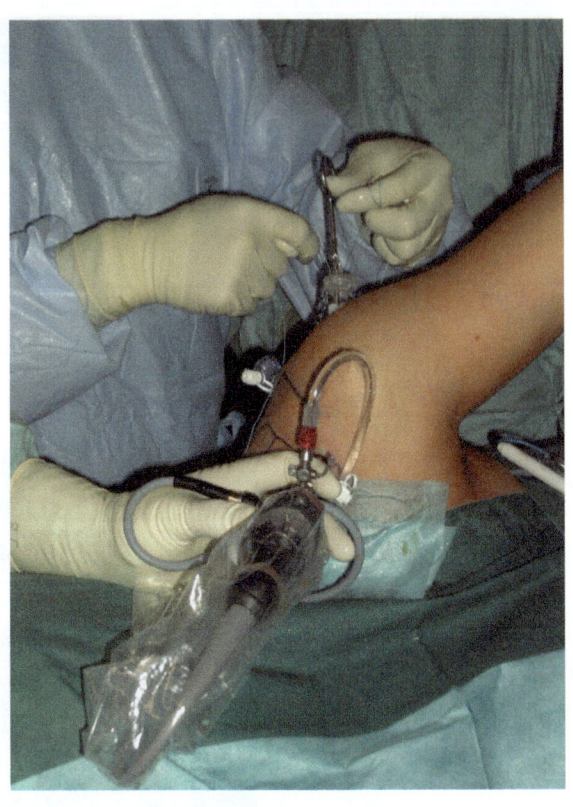

Fig. 8.13 Reconstructed
labrum

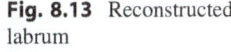

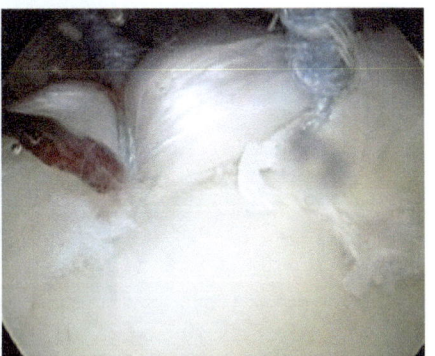

3. Open reposition or osteosynthesis of glenoid fractures.
4. Open posteroinferior capsular shift.

Indications for open procedure include:

• Pathologic retroversion of the glenoid → osteotomy of the glenoid.

- Bony defects of the glenoid or glenoidal erosion → posterior bone block procedure.
- Big "reversed" bony Bankart or glenoid fracture → reposition or osteosynthesis of glenoid rim fractures.
- Recurrent posterior instability (failed arthroscopic procedure).

Usually a routine diagnostic arthroscopy is performed with every surgical procedure. In cases where open procedure is definitely we prefer prone position for better exposure of the glenohumeral joint and the glenoid plane.

The skin is incised vertical 7–10 cm parallel to the glenohumeral joint starting from below the superior scapula spine directed to the axillary fold. The deltoid fascia is cut in-line with the muscle fibers and the deltoid muscle is split. Blunt deep retractors are placed and the infraspinatus and the teres minor muscles are exposed and identified by rotating the arm. Both muscles are covered by a solid fascia that needs to be cut in line with the muscle fibres. The suprascapular nerve runs approximately 1.5 cm medially to the glenoid rim, so the incision starting from the lateral tendinous portion of the infraspinatus has to be performed carefully. In order to access the capsule the infraspinatus is retracted and elevated. Due to the short tendinous insertion of the infraspinatus and its attachment to the capsule it has to be split laterally.

A T-shape capsular incision is performed by a primary vertical cut at the glenoid side to keep sufficient stock for later capsular shifting. The longitudinal incision is placed right above the pIGHL. The two flaps get marked with sutures and retracted for exposition of the joint.

In case of a posterior labral lesion a refixation with suture anchors is performed. The glenoid rim is debrided and the posterior labrum is mobilized thoroughly. As in the arthroscopic procedure we suggest placing the most inferior suture anchor first.

A capsular shift is performed in a pants over vest fashion bringing the inferior capsular flap superiorly. The superior part of the capsular flap is sutured posteroinferiorly over the inferior flap either using the sutures of the anchors or additional stitches. After closing the lower recessus with of the anchor sutures, the lower capsular flap can be fixed to the upper one in an overlapping way in approximately 45° abducted position. Additionally both flaps are secured with backup sutures.

Pathologic glenoid retroversion of ≥ 15–$20°$ can cause recurrent posterior instability and indicates surgical correction by means of open wedge osteotomy because isolated soft tissue procedures can not adequately restore posterior stability of the shoulder.

For proper exposure of the glenoid the posterior capsule needs sufficient medial mobilization. A blunt instrument or retractor is introduced into the joint space to mark the glenoid plane. Subsequently two K-wires are placed about 5 mm medial and parallel to the joint line to prevent fracturing the glenoid face while performing the osteotomy of the posterior cortex with a sharp osteotome right medial to the K-wires. The 2–3 cm wedge shaped bone graft can be harvested either from the iliac crest or the postero-superior spine of the scapula. For better inhealing the graft is cleaned of soft tissue and carefully decorticated with a burr. Fixation of the graft is press-fit and usually does not require screws. The joint capsule is closed covering the bone graft in the above described pants-over-vest fashion.

In patients with bony defects or glenoid erosions a corticospongious span can recreate the posterior glenoid rim.

Scott [44] described an operative procedure with a graft harvested from the spine of the scapula that is screw-fixated to the posteroinferior sector of the glenoid.

Another option is to use Resch's press-fit J-Span [45] at the posteriorly bone deficient glenoid.

Wound closing is done in layers in the usual fashion. The arm is placed in an abduction orthesis with 0° rotation.

8.5   Postoperative Rehabilitation

Physical therapy starts the day after surgery. Patients are carefully instructed in the adequate behavior and precautions to protect the operative reconstruction. The abduction orthesis is advised for 6 weeks.

Within the first 3 weeks postoperatively active-assisted abduction up to 45° is permitted, passive flexion up to 30°, internal rotation up to 30° an external rotation up to 60°. From week 4–6 abduction can be preceded to 90°, internal and external rotation to 45 and 75° respectively. By week 9 unlimited range of motion is allowed. Besides mobilizing the shoulder thoroughly, strengthening of the rotator cuff and improvement of the scapular setting are performed.

8.6   Outcomes

According to the literature arthroscopic treatment of posterior instability achieves success rates between 88 and 92 % at a follow-up of at least 2 years [46, 47]. Savoie [48] even published a success rate of 97 % using the Neer-Foster rating system. Compared to the results of arthroscopic treatment of anterior instability the outcomes of posterior stabilization are described to be not as excellent [2, 3, 8, 11, 48, 49]. A major reason may be the fact that unlike in anterior instability the etiology appears to be more complex [48]. Successful open surgical treatment of posterior shoulder instability is reported in the literature with good to excellent results of 75–91 % and a recurrence rate of 7–30 % [3, 28, 33, 50, 51]. Graichen [52] reported an instability recurrence rate of 12.5 % at a 5 years follow-up, but concomitant osteoarthritis after open-wedge osteotomy of the glenoid. Servien [35] published comparable results for a posterior bone block procedure.

8.7 Summary

Diagnostics and surgical treatment of posterior shoulder instability is still challenging. But this relatively rare condition can be reliably diagnosed with raised awareness of the pathology and better understanding of shoulder biomechanics. So far in literature there is still controversy about the individual contribution of the varying mechanical factors, as some are also present in asymptomatic patients. If conservative management fails, surgical intervention offers various surgical options to address individual pathologies depending on the patients' symptoms, x-ray, MRI and CT scans as well as on a thorough clinical exam under anesthesia and diagnostic arthroscopy.

In the past arthroscopic procedures became more advanced with reliable postoperative outcomes, but still special pathologies need open surgical proceedings.

References

1. Ahlgren SA, Hedlund T, Nistor L (1978) Idiopathic posterior instability of the shoulder joint. Results of operation with posterior bone graft. Acta Orthopaedica Scandinavica 49:600–603
2. Antoniou J, Duckworth DT, Harryman DT 2nd (2000) Capsulolabral augmentation for the the management of posteroinferior instability of the shoulder. Am J Bone Joint Surg 82:1220–1230
3. Bottoni CR, Franks BR, Moore JH et al (2005) Operative stabilization of posterior shoulder instability. Am J Sports Med 33:996–1002
4. Boyd HB, Sisk TD (1972) Recurrent posterior dislocation of the shoulder. Am J Bone Joint Surg 54:779–786
5. Goubier JN, Iserin A, Duranthon LD et al. (2003) A 4-portal arthroscopic stabilization in posterior shoulder instability. J Shoulder Elbow Surg Am Shoulder Elbow Surg... [et al] 12:337–341
6. Mc Laughlin H (1952) Posterior dislocation of the shoulder. Am J Bone Joint Surg 24-A-3:584–590
7. Owens BD, Duffey ML, Nelson BJ et al (2007) The incidence and characteristics of shoulder instability at the United States Military Academy. Am J Sports Med 35:1168–1173
8. Provencher MT, Bell SJ, Menzel KA et al (2005) Arthroscopic treatment of posterior shoulder instability: results in 33 patients. Am J Sports Med 33:1463–1471
9. Provencher MT, Leclere LE, King S et al (2011) Posterior instability of the shoulder: diagnosis and management. Am J Sports Med 39:874–886
10. Robinson CM, Seah M, Akhtar MA (2011) The epidemiology, risk of recurrence, and functional outcome after an acute traumatic posterior dislocation of the shoulder. Am J Bone Joint Surg 93:1605–1613
11. Wolf EM, Eakin CL (1998) Arthroscopic capsular plication for posterior shoulder instability. J Arthrosc Relat Surg 14:153–163
12. Neer CS 2nd (1985) Involuntary inferior and multidirectional instability of the shoulder: etiology, recognition, and treatment. Instr Course Lect 34:232–238
13. Feely Bt MC (2011) Posterior Shoulder Stabilization. In: Fu FH (ed) Master technique in orthopaedic surgery sports medicine. Lippincott Williams & Wilkins, Philadelphia
14. Bey MJ, Hunter SA, Kilambi N et al. (2005) Structural and mechanical properties of the glenohumeral Joint posterior capsule. J Shoulder Elbow Surg Am Shoulder Elbow Surg... [et al] 14:201–206

15. Lintner SA, Levy A, Kenter K et al (1996) Glenohumeral translation in the asymptomatic athlete's shoulder and its relationship to other clinically measurable anthropometric variables. Am J Sports Med 24:716–720

16. O'connell PW, Nuber GW, Mileski RA et al (1990) The contribution of the glenohumeral ligaments to anterior stability of the shoulder joint. Am J Sports Med 18:579–584

17. Turkel SJ, Panio MW, Marshall JL et al (1981) Stabilizing mechanisms preventing anterior dislocation of the glenohumeral joint. Am J Bone Joint Surg 63:1208–1217

18. Dewing CB, Mccormick F, Bell SJ et al (2008) An analysis of capsular area in patients with anterior, posterior, and multidirectional shoulder instability. Am J Sports Med 36:515–522

19. Kim SH, Noh KC, Park JS et al (2005) Loss of chondrolabral containment of the glenohumeral Jt in atraumatic posteroinferior multidirectional instability. Am J Bone Joint Surg 87:92–98

20. Matsen FA 3rd, Chebli C, Lippitt S et al (2006) Principles for the evaluation and management of shoulder instability. Am J Bone Joint Surg 88:648–659

21. Lévigne C (2008) Classification of posterior shoulder instability. In: Boileau P (ed) Shoulder concepts. Sauramps medical, Montpellier

22. Lichtenberg S, Habermeyer P (2009) Open and arthroscopic procedures for posterior shoulder instability. Der Orthopade 38:54–63

23. Robinson CM, Aderinto J (2005) Recurrent posterior shoulder instability. Am J Bone Joint Surg 87:883–892

24. Bradley JP, Forsythe B, Mascarenhas R (2008) Arthroscopic management of posterior shoulder instability: diagnosis, indications, and technique. Clin Sports Med 27:649–670

25. Millett PJ, Clavert P, Hatch GF 3rd et al (2006) Recurrent posterior shoulder instability. J Am Acad Orthop Surg 14:464–476

26. Fuchs B, Jost B, Gerber C (2000) Posterior-inferior capsular shift for the treatment of recurrent, voluntary posterior subluxation of the shoulder. Am J Bone Joint Surg 82:16–25

27. Burkhead WZ Jr, Rockwood CA Jr (1992) Treatment of instability of the shoulder with an exercise program. Am J Bone Joint Surg 74:890–896

28. Fronek J, Warren RF, Bowen M (1989) Posterior subluxation of the glenohumeral joint. Am J Bone Joint Surg 71:205–216

29. Schwartz E, Warren RF, O'brien SJ et al (1987) Posterior shoulder instability. Orthop Clin North Am 18:409–419

30. Hawkins RJ, Koppert G, Johnston G (1984) Recurrent posterior instability (subluxation) of the shoulder. Am J Bone Joint Surg 66:169–174

31. Lenart BA, Sherman SL, Mall NA et al (2012) Arthroscopic repair for posterior shoulder instability. Arthroscopy J Arthrosc Relat Surg 28:1337–1343

32. Pollock RG, Bigliani LU (1993) Recurrent posterior shoulder instability. Diagnosis and treatment. Clinical Orthop Relat Res 291:85–96

33. Wolf BR, Strickland S, Williams RJ et al (2005) Open posterior stabilization for recurrent posterior glenohumeral instability. J Shoulder Elbow Surg Am Shoulder Elbow Surg... [et al] 14:157–164

34. Hawkins RH (1996) Glenoid osteotomy for recurrent posterior subluxation of the shoulder: assessment by computed axial tomography. J Shoulder Elbow Surg Am Shoulder Elbow Surg... [et al] 5:393–400

35. Servien E, Walch G, Cortes ZE et al (2007) Posterior bone block procedure for posterior shoulder instability. Knee Surg Sports Traumatol Arthrosc 15:1130–1136

36. Cofield RH, Irving JF (1987) Evaluation and classification of shoulder instability. With special reference to examination under anesthesia. Clin Orthop Relat Res 223:32–43

37. Blasier RB, Soslowsky LJ, Malicky DM et al (1997) Posterior glenohumeral subluxation: active and passive stabilization in a biomechanical model. Am J Bone Joint Surg 79:433–440

38. Kim SH, Park JS, Jeong WK et al (2005) The Kim test: a novel test for posteroinferior labral lesion of the shoulder—a comparison to the jerk test. Am J Sports Med 33:1188–1192

39. Gerber C, Ganz R (1984) Clinical assessment of instability of the shoulder. With special reference to anterior and posterior drawer tests. Br J Bone Joint Surg 66:551–556
40. Hewitt M, Getelman MH, Snyder SJ (2003) Arthroscopic management of multidirectional instability: pancapsular plication. Orthop Clin North Am 34:549–557
41. Lichtenberg S, Habermeyer P, Magosch P (2007) Arthroscopic treatment of posterior shoulder instability. Operative Orthopadie und Traumatologie 19:115–132
42. Gerber C, Ganz R, Vinh TS (1987) Glenoplasty for recurrent posterior shoulder instability. An anatomic reappraisal. Clin Orthop Relat Res 216:70–79
43. Karas SG, Creighton RA, Demorat GJ (2004) Glenohumeral volume reduction in arthroscopic shoulder reconstruction: a cadaveric analysis of suture plication and thermal capsulorrhaphy. J Arthrosc Relat Surg 20:179–184
44. Scott DJ Jr (1967) Treatment of recurrent posterior dislocations of the shoulder by glenoplasty. Report of three cases. Am J Bone Joint Surg 49:471–476
45. Auffarth A, Schauer J, Matis N et al (2008) The J-bone graft for anatomical glenoid reconstruction in recurrent posttraumatic anterior shoulder dislocation. Am J Sports Med 36:638–647
46. Bradley JP, Baker CL 3rd, Kline AJ et al (2006) Arthroscopic capsulolabral reconstruction for posterior instability of the shoulder: a prospective study of 100 shoulders. Am J Sports Med 34:1061–1071
47. Williams RJ 3rd, Strickland S, Cohen M et al (2003) Arthroscopic repair for traumatic posterior shoulder instability. Am J Sports Med 31:203–209
48. Savoie FH 3rd, Holt MS, Field LD et al (2008) Arthroscopic management of posterior instability: evolution of technique and results. J Arthrosc Relat Surg 24:389–396
49. Radkowski CA, Chhabra A, Baker CL 3rd et al (2008) Arthroscopic capsulolabral repair for posterior shoulder instability in throwing athletes compared with nonthrowing athletes. Am J Sports Med 36:693–699
50. Tibone J, Ting A (1990) Capsulorrhaphy with a staple for recurrent posterior subluxation of the shoulder. Am J Bone Joint Surg 72:999–1002
51. Tibone JE, Bradley JP (1993) The treatment of posterior subluxation in athletes. Clin Orthop Relat Res 291:124–137
52. Graichen H, Koydl P, Zichner L (1998) Value of glenoid osteotomy in treatment of posterior shoulder instability. Zeitschrift fur Orthopadie und ihre Grenzgebiete 136:238–242

Management of SLAP Lesions: Where are We in 2013?

9

Mark Sando, R. Frank Henn and Stephen R. Thompson

9.1 Introduction

Tears of the superior glenoid labrum were first described by Andrews and colleagues in 1985. Evaluation of 73 overhead throwing athletes found that 83 % of labral tears were in the anterosuperior region at the biceps tendon/labrum complex [1]. In 1990, Synder et al. recognized a similar type of superior labral injury and were the first to categorize and classify these lesions. They also named the injury a superior labrum anterior and posterior (SLAP) lesion [2]. Since that time, numerous studies have sought to identify the pertinent anatomy, pathophysiology, diagnostic criterion, and appropriate treatment methods of SLAP lesions.

The true incidence of SLAP lesions in the overall population is unknown. Synder identified a 6 % incidence amongst 2375 patients undergoing arthroscopic evaluation [3]. Percentage rates have varied in other reports, however, the current literature maintains that this is a relatively uncommon injury. A low incidence, as well as a lack of consensus surrounding the need for surgical repair, debridement or biceps tenodesis has made operative management of SLAP lesions a controversial topic [4, 5]. Despite this, overall rates for surgical repair of these lesions have remained high compared with incidence, with recent literature suggesting the

Disclosures: The authors did not receive any outside funding or grants in support of their research for or preparation of this work. Neither they nor a member of their immediate families received payments or other benefits or a commitment or agreement to provide such benefits from a commercial entity.

M. Sando · R. F. Henn
Department of Orthopaedics, University of Maryland, Baltimore, MD, USA

S. R. Thompson (✉)
Fowler-Kennedy Sport Medicine Clinic 3 M-Centre, University of Western Ontario, London, ON N6A 3K7, Canada
e-mail: theskip@gmail.com

S. F. Brockmeier et al. (eds.), *Surgery of Shoulder Instability*, DOI: 10.1007/978-3-642-38100-3_9, © ISAKOS 2013

frequency of repair is on the rise [6, 7]. Weber et al. analyzed 4975 cases of SLAP repairs collected from the American Board of Orthopaedic Surgery (ABOS) Boards Part II and found that ABOS candidates were performing SLAP repairs at a rate 3 times higher than expected based on epidemiologic data [6]. The age of patients undergoing repair was also higher than expected with average age of males being 37, and females being 40, with reported cases of 85 and 88 year old patients undergoing SLAP repair [6].

The controversy surrounding proper management of these lesions stems from the lack of quality evidence currently available. A systematic review of the literature regarding repair of type II SLAP lesions found that there is currently no level I or II evidence for isolated SLAP repair outcomes [8]. The data available shows a range of good to excellent outcomes of 40–94 %. A prospective, level III study by Boileau et al. compared the outcomes of type II SLAP repair versus biceps tenodesis and found significantly better results in the tenodesis group in regards to subjective satisfaction and return to play [5]. These results, however, were based on only 25 patients who were not randomized. The lack of prospective, randomized outcome measures has furthered the controversy and has led to a large variation in treatment algorithms [4].

So where do we stand in 2013 on the issues of understanding, diagnosing and treating SLAP tears? The purpose of this review is to provide an update on SLAP tears and their management based on the best evidence currently available.

9.2 Anatomy

The key to diagnosing and understanding SLAP tears is a full understanding of the anatomy of the superior glenoid labrum and biceps tendon complex. A recent anatomic study by Bain confirmed several key features of the superior labral complex that are crucial for understanding its function as a partial restraint to antero-inferior translation of the humeral head, and in providing torsional rigidity to the abducted, externally rotated shoulder. The superior labrum is concave and has a loose, mobile interface that may attach to the glenoid rim, but more commonly attaches medially, off of the glenoid face. The long head of the biceps tendon consistently attaches to the supraglenoid tubercle, 6.6 mm from the glenoid face at the 12 o'clock position. While the tendon is histologically discrete, approximately one third of the fibers are attached to the superior labrum. There is also a consistent synovial recess between the superior labrum and biceps tendon that should not be confused with a pathologic lesion. This recess occurs between the biceps tendon fibers inserting into the labrum and those inserting into the tubercle and is a separate entity from any sublabral foramen that are found between the labrum and articular cartilage surface. These sublabral foramen or recesses are most commonly found between 12 and 3 o'clock position in a right shoulder and do not extend posterior to the biceps insertion; anything outside of this zone is likely pathologic [9].

This recent study confirms classic findings of Vangsness who found that approximately 50 % of biceps tendon fibers attached to the superior labrum and 50 % to the supraglenoid tubercle [10]. He also observed four types of biceps tendon attachments including: type I—an entirely posterior labral attachment (22 %), type II—a mostly posterior labral attachment (33 %), type III—equal anterior and posterior labral attachments (37 %) and type IV—an entirely anterior labral attachment (8 %) [10].

The idea of a mobile superior glenoid as a normal anatomic variant is also supported by the arthroscopic findings of Davidson and Rivenburgh. They identified a group of 49 patients with articular cartilage on the supraglenoid tubercle, a mobile labrum, and no evidence of injury or fraying [11]. A cadaveric, histologic analysis by Podromos et al. found however firm attachments of the labrum to the glenoid rim in all specimens under the age of 30. There was detachment of the labrum from the glenoid rim, predominantly in the anterosuperior zone in 4/17 patients older than 36 at time of death [12]. This brings into question whether or not the concept of a loose, mobile superior labrum is a normal anatomic variant or a result of aging and degenerative change.

The superior labrum is typically triangular in shape, however anatomic variants exist. Davidson described three variants including a triangular labrum, a bumper labrum that abuts the articular margin and is firmly attached to the rim, and a meniscoid labrum with the free edge draped over the articular surface [11]. The labrum may attach directly to the glenoid rim but more commonly it attaches medial to it creating a sublabral recess. Cadaveric analyses by Smith et al. and Waldt et al. confirm the presence of a sublabral recess, or foramen, as an "anatomic variant" in 73 and 74 % of specimens, respectively [13, 14]. Smith describes 4 types of superior labral attachment including: type I—firm attachment, no recess; type II—recess less than 2 mm deep; type II—recess greater than 2 mm, but less than 5 mm deep; type IV—recess greater than 5 mm deep. They also observed a higher prevalence of type III and IV labral attachments in patients older than 66 years, again questioning the sublabral recess as a normal variant versus degenerative change. Comparative MR arthrograms of these cadaver specimens led Smith to conclude that the sublabral recess is a common normal variant existing between the superior glenoid rim and the anterior half of the superior labrum, but does not extend posterior to the biceps tendon origin [13].

Other notable anatomic variants include sublabral foramen, sublabral foramen with a thickened middle glenohumeral ligament (9 % of shoulders) and the Buford complex, defined as an absent anterosuperior labrum with a thickened middle glenohumeral ligament (1.5 % of shoulders) [4]. Recognition of these variants is important as they do not necessitate treatment, and attempted repair with attachment of the MGHL to the glenoid rim may lead to external rotation deficits.

Osseous anatomy of the glenoid is also variable and may have an effect on labral pathology. It has been suggested that an increase in glenoid retroversion may be protective against SLAP lesions [15]. It has been postulated that overhead throwers who undergo morphologic changes to glenoid anatomy, including increased retroversion, as well as increased humeral retrotorsion place less stress on the superolabral/biceps tendon complex. The evidence for this however is level IV and needs to be followed up with better prospective analysis and anatomic evaluation.

9.3   Classification

Retrospective review of over 700 shoulder arthroscopies by Synder et al. led to the identification and classification of this injury pattern into 4 types, with this remaining as the prominent classification system to date [2].

Type I describes superior labral fraying and degeneration with maintenance of the labral/biceps anchor attachment. Type II (the most common type) refers to a detachment of the superior labral/biceps anchor complex from the glenoid. Type III lesions result in a bucket handle tear of the labrum with an intact biceps anchor attachment. The displaced labral fragment may produce mechanical symptoms if displaced into the glenohumeral joint. Type IV describes a bucket handle tear that extends into the biceps tendon, creating a split in the tendon with some portion usually remaining attached to the glenoid [2]. The amount of the biceps tendon involved dictates treatment.

The initial classification scheme has since been expanded. Type II has been broken down into IIa—primarily anterior detachment of labral/biceps complex, IIb—primarily posterior detachment of labral/biceps complex, and IIc—combined anterior and posterior detachment [16]. Maffet further described three additional variants with antero-inferior extension including: type V: SLAP tear combined with a Bankart lesion, type VI—SLAP tear combined with unstable flap tear of the labrum, and type VII—SLAP tear with continuation to the MGHL origin [17]. While the Synder classification system remains the most commonly used, there is a significant amount of inter and intraobserver variability in the diagnosis and treatment of SLAP tears based on this system [18].

9.4   Principles of Diagnosis

The diagnosis of SLAP tears is often challenging due to variations in patient history, inconsistent physical exam findings, and difficulty in interpreting imaging results. It is often said that the true diagnosis can only be made at time of arthroscopy however wide interobserver and intraobserver variability exists here as well [4, 18, 19]. The key to proper diagnosis involves a careful history, methodical examination, and interpretation of radiographic findings.

Patient history is often variable, but is critical in identifying a particular mechanism likely to cause SLAP lesions. The history usually consists of a traction, compression, or repetitive overhead throwing mechanism. Patients may report an episode of shoulder instability or dislocation with traction or compression injuries. Insidious onset is frequently reported, especially in overuse injuries seen in overhead throwing athletes. Pain is the primary complaint, along with mechanical symptoms of "catching" or "popping" with activity. The location of pain is highly variable and can be posterior, postero-superior, anterosuperior, or referred to the bicipital groove.

In his initial observation, Andrews reported that the contraction of the biceps muscle leads to tightening of the long head tendon and raises the superior labrum off the glenoid rim. He theorized that these forces imparted from the biceps tendon onto the superior labrum during the follow through phase of throwing lead to the anterosuperior labral tears [1].

In contrast Synder described a mechanism of falls onto outstretched hands in the flexed and abducted position leading to compression of the glenohumeral joint. They hypothesized that the compressive force on the joint, as well as proximal humeral head migration led to a pinching of the superior labrum/biceps tendon complex causing traumatic disruption. Arm position at time of pinching thus led to migration of the tear and variation in patterns [2].

Another described mechanism of injury is due to traction, usually an inferiorly directed force. Maffet et al. found this to be the predominant mechanism of injury in a study of 712 patients undergoing arthroscopic shoulder procedures [17]. This study found that 38 % of patients with superior labral tears had further extension in an anteroinferior direction and thus did not fit into the 4 types initially described by Snyder. This lead to the addition of types V and VI to the classification system [17].

While Andrews described a tensile failure of the labral complex at the biceps anchor, Burkhart et al. have suggested a torsional failure known as the "peel-back" mechanism [20]. In this model, during the cocking phase of throwing with the arm in the abducted and externally rotated position, the biceps force vector shifts to a more posterior and vertically oriented direction. This creates a torsional load at the base of the biceps that rotates the posterior labrum and biceps tendon medially over the corner of the glenoid. This "peel-back" phenomenon is then repeated with every overhead throwing motion and can propagate a posterior directed SLAP lesion.

Once a proper history is elucidated, physical exam becomes the next component of diagnosis. Unfortunately, a reliable physical exam test to diagnosis SLAP tears does not exist [4]. Numerous maneuvers have been described, however the current recommendation is that these be used in concert, along with a proper patient history [21].

Some of the provocative tests commonly utilized include: O'Brien test, compression-rotation test, Speed test, dynamic labral shear test, Kibler anterior slide test, crank test, and the Kim biceps load test. A systematic review of available literature analyzing the validity of the numerous provocative tests found that poor study methodology has made it difficult to draw any conclusions regarding diagnostic accuracy [22]. Cook et al. performed a diagnostic study utilizing five tests: O'Brien's, Kim biceps load test, Speed test, Dynamic labral shear test, and the labral tension test. None of these tests demonstrated diagnostic utility as stand alone or clustered tests in diagnosing SLAP lesions in patients with arthroscopically confirmed tears [23]. It is important to note however that there is controversy regarding these findings, as the dynamic labral shear test was not performed in the manner initially described by O'Driscoll et al. and reproduced by Kibler [24–26]. These initial studies found a sensitivity of 0.86, and a likelihood ratio of 31.57 for the dyanamic labral shear test for labral injury [26]. With varying reports on reliability of the numerous provocative maneuvers, the concept of "the suspicious exam" proposed by Burns and Synder seems most relevant in decision making to pursue further diagnostic modalities. This approach relies on the proper patient described mechanism of injury, symptoms, and one or more positive provocative tests leading to a suspicion that should be validated with imaging.

Magnetic resonance imaging remains the hallmark of SLAP diagnosis. MRI findings consistent with type II SLAP tears include high signal intensity extension under the superior labrum/biceps root on coronal images (Fig. 9.1).

Antero-posterior extension of high signal intensity at the labral/biceps root on axial images is also suggestive of SLAP tear. A paralabral cyst is indicative of a labral tear, and a cyst arising from a SLAP tear may extend to the spinoglenoid notch and compress the suprascapular nerve. The question of whether or not conventional MRI is adequate to diagnose SLAP tears or if MR arthrography is required has been addressed. Phillips et al. found that non-contrast MRIs were not helpful in diagnosing isolated SLAP lesions or SLAP lesions with concomitant injuries. Non-contrast MRI had a sensitivity of 86 %, but a specificity of only 13 %, while the post-test probability of both positive and negative findings resulted in decision-making that was worse than if the MRI was not obtained [27]. MR arthrograms are reported to be much more accurate in diagnosing SLAP tears. A direct comparison of noncontrast MRI and MR arthrography by Amin and

Fig. 9.1 T2 weighted coronal MRI scan demonstrating increased signal under and within the superior labrum

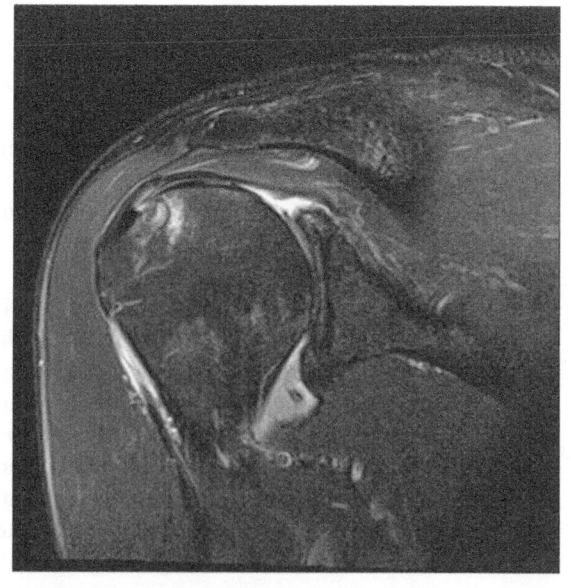

Yousseff found that of 34 patients diagnosed with normal MRI, 22 were found to have SLAP tears on MR arthrography. The MRA was found to be 90 % sensitive, 50 % specific and correlated to arthroscopy results in 79.3 % of patients [28]. Though not perfect, MR arthrography improves diagnosis and can especially help to avoid unnecessary arthroscopy when negative in a patient with equivocal or non-specific physical examination findings.

Diagnosis of SLAP tears remains a challenging task, even to the most skilled physician. A careful elucidation of the patient's mechanism of injury, specific symptoms, and combination of provocative maneuvers must be utilized. A "suspicious exam" based on careful observation should lead to further imaging [4]. Standard radiographs are of course important to eliminate other pathology, but MR arthrogram is the test of choice for evaluating labral pathology. An MR arthrogram negative for labral pathology is highly suggestive of another etiology and without other positive findings should lead to a treatment plan of observation and physiotherapy. MR arthrogram suggestive of a SLAP tear should lead to a discussion of further treatment.

9.5 Principles of Treatment

Management of SLAP lesions is controversial, Nonoperative management should be initially attempted in virtually all patients. The goals of rehabilitation should focus on alleviating symptoms and addressing concurrent pathology. Physiotherapy should be directed at rotator cuff strengthening and scapular stabilization to improve mechanics. For most overhead throwers, improving flexibility of the posterior capsule is also recommended. Intra-articular injections may be of both diagnostic and therapeutic benefit and may help progress therapy by reducing pain. Edwards et al. demonstrated successful non-operative management in a group of patients with isolated SLAP tears who at an average of 3.1 years follow-up had improved pain relief and functional outcome scores when compared to pre-treatment. 71 % of athletes treated non-operatively returned to pre-participation levels, but only 66 % of overhead throwing athletes [29]. The authors concluded that in overhead athletes and in patients where rehabilitation fails to provide relief or improve symptoms, surgical management should be considered.

Once a decision is made that non-operative management has failed and surgical treatment is recommended the next decision the surgeon faces is to proceed with arthroscopic repair of the SLAP tear versus debridement and biceps tenodesis. There is some agreement that older patients with obvious biceps pathology and degenerative labral tearing or fraying are best treated with debridement and biceps tenodesis [4]. In younger patients, type I tears are typically treated with minimal debridement. Type III tears are generally treated with resection of the unstable labral fragment and possible repair of the MGHL if it is attached to the torn fragment. Type IV tears are generally treated with debridement alone when less than 30 % of the biceps tendon is involved, and labral repair or debridement (depending upon patient age) and biceps tenodesis when greater than 30 % of the tendon is involved [30].

Controversy surrounds management of type II SLAP tears. Boileau et al. observed improved Constant scores and patient satisfaction in patients treated with biceps tenodesis (80 % satisfaction) compared with SLAP repair (40 % satisfaction). They also reported an improved return to pre-participation activity with tenodesis versus repair. However, it is important to note that the mean age of the repair group was 15 years younger than the tenodesis group [5]. While there is a definite role for biceps tenodesis as an effective treatment of SLAP tears, there is not current evidence available to apply this strategy to all ages and activity levels.

Numerous approaches exist for repairing type II SLAP tears. Unfortunately, to date, there remains little evidence to suggest superiority of any precise repair configuration. Suture anchors in the glenoid rim along with simple or mattress sutures are most commonly employed. Common suture anchor configurations include one or two suture anchors posterior to the biceps anchor, two anchors with one anterior and one posterior, and a single suture anchor centrally placed with suture through the biceps origin [31] or on either side of the tendon in a "nonstrangulating" fashion [4].

Biomechanical studies comparing these configurations have presented conflicting data with one suggesting higher strain to failure with a mattress suture through the biceps origin, while another found no difference between two posterior anchors and one anterior, one posterior anchor configurations [31, 32]. Similarly it is unclear if a mattress suture technique versus a simple suture configuration is clinically important. In a cadaver model, Boddula et al. found that a mattress suture significantly increased labral height compared with the native tissue, theoretically creating a bumper effect. The mattress sutured labrum did experience a higher strain indicating that it held more firm, and the labrum was observed to "slip" under the simple suture construct. This however did not provide any improved biomechanical advantage compared with the simple suture [33]. Conclusive data on preferred repair constructs is still lacking.

Concomitant pathology can also affect the treatment algorithm. In overhead throwing athletes, the presence of a partial thickness rotator cuff tear has been shown to have a negative effect on clinical outcomes after SLAP repair alone [34]. Concurrent rotator cuff repair in addition to SLAP repair has shown good clinical outcomes [16]. However, Kim et al. found that patients undergoing RTC repair and biceps tenotomy had improved functional shoulder scores and range of motion at 2 year follow-up compared with RTC repair and SLAP repair [35]. The average age of patients in these groups however were 63 and 61, respectively, and the patients were not randomized. Two randomized studies have demonstrated that there is no advantage to repairing a SLAP at the time of rotator cuff repair in patients older than 45 and 50 years [36, 37].

9.6   Authors Preferred SLAP Repair Technique

We utilize the standard posterior viewing portal and the standard 5 mm anterior interval portal. A standard diagnostic arthroscopy is performed and the extent of the tear is assessed. An anterolateral interval working portal is placed superior to the biceps using needle localization. The portal is dilated and a 7 mm cannula is inserted. The labrum is debrided and the superior glenoid rim is abraded to create a bony bed for healing. The extent of the tear is reassessed and anchor placement is planned. For Type IIA tears, a single biocomposite labral anchor is placed just posterior to the biceps at 1130 to 12 O'Clock in a right shoulder through the anterolateral interval portal. For more posterior tears, a percutaneous portal of Wilmington is utilized for anchor placement to minimize risk of injury to the suprascapular nerve during anchor placement. After needle localization, a sharp trocar is utilized to introduce the anchor drill guide without a cannula through the myotendinous junction of the rotator cuff. We believe this minimizes rotator cuff trauma. Sutures are shuttled using a curved suture passer via the anterolateral portal. Knots are tied through the anterolateral cannula. We prefer simple sutures with the knot on the capsular side (Fig. 9.2a, b). We rarely place anchors anterior to the biceps origin due to concern for over constraining the biceps and increasing the risk of stiffness.

9.7   Outcomes

Recent literature suggests good to excellent outcomes at greater than 5 year follow-up. Denard et al. found that patients over 40 reported fewer good to excellent results than those under 40 (81 % vs. 97 %) though this did not reach statistical significance. Patients receiving worker's compensation did significantly worse, with only 65 % good to excellent outcomes compared with 95 % good to excellent outcomes in non-compensation patients [38]. In a group of Norwegian patients,

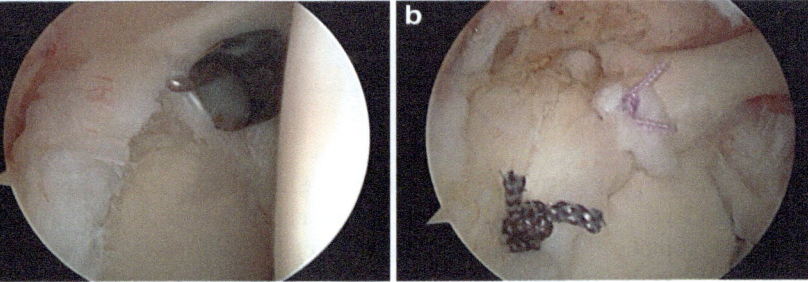

Fig. 9.2 a Arthroscopic image of a Type II SLAP lesion viewed from the posterior portal. Detachment and increased mobility of the superior labrum at the root of the biceps anchor is noted. **b** Same lesion after repair using two suture anchors posterior to the biceps

Schroder found 88 % good to excellent results at 5 year follow-up with no significant difference between patients over and under 40 years of age. Eighty-three percent of patients also reported returning to pre-injury level of activity [39]. Other literature with shorter follow-up similarly suggests good clinical results in patients over 40, and that isolated SLAP repairs in older patients do better than combined SLAP and RTC repairs [40].

A systematic review of literature with a minimum of 2 year follow up concluded that for type II SLAP repairs, excellent outcomes can largely be expected for patients not involved in throwing or overhead sports [8]. When focusing on athletes, a review of 14 studies undertaken by Sayde et al. found good to excellent patient satisfaction in 83 % with 73 % returning to previous level of play at a minimum of 2-year follow-up [41]. Only 63 % of overhead athletes however returned to pre-injury level of play. This review also noted improved outcomes in repairs performed with suture anchors over those with bioabsorbable tacks, reflecting the current trend in practice [41]. The diminished outcomes in overhead throwers are fairly consistent throughout the current literature in functional outcomes, subjective assessment, and return to play [42, 43]. Brockmeier et al. interestingly found improved patient satisfaction outcomes and return to prior competition level in athletes reporting a specific traumatic etiology to their injury versus those with more insidious onset [43].

Not surprisingly, patients undergoing revision procedures for failed repair predictably perform worse. In a retrospective review of 12 patients who underwent revision SLAP repair, Park and Glousman found that pain was the chief complaint at both initial and revision surgery. Compared to after initial surgery, mean return to work was 57.8 % and mean return to sports was 42 % of the previous level. None of the four baseball players returned to play and patients receiving worker's compensation had lower outcome data [44].

Pain after SLAP repair may be multifactorial and is rarely caused by simple failure. Revision of failed SLAP repair requires special attention and pre-operative workup to elucidate the true cause. In instances of true repair failure, a re-repair can be attempted, but literature suggests likely better results with debridement and biceps tenotomy or tenodesis in patients over 40 or with any biceps damage [4, 5, 45]. Further study is necessary to know if this approach will yield better results in a younger patient population.

9.8 Complications

While becoming increasingly more common, SLAP repair is not a benign procedure and comes with risk of both intra- and post-operative complications. Reported complications include iatrogenic rotator cuff tears, persistent pain, stiffness, loosening or migration of implants leading to synovitis or arthritis, and suprascapular nerve injury [45–47]. As the prevalence of SLAP repair increases, it is becoming evident that these complications have long-term effects and are likely more common than initially thought with a surgeon reported rate of 4.4 % [7].

The most common post-operative complication reported is stiffness. Careful assessment of passive range of motion is critical, as well as recognizing concomitant pathology [45]. Katz et al. evaluated 39 patients presenting with problems after SLAP repair and found 75 % with a chief complaint of pain and limited range of motion. All patients with limited range of motion were treated initially with physical therapy with 29 % reporting improved outcome to good or excellent after conservative treatment alone. Of the remaining patients who were unhappy with conservative management, most had achieved acceptable range of motion with therapy but still had pain [46]. The patients in this review were also older (average age 43), and 50 % were receiving worker's compensation. This highlights the complex etiology of "failed" SLAP repair as a multifactorial entity. Patients with improved range of motion with conservative management need to be assessed for other underlying pathology as the source of pain. Those with restricted ROM that does not improve are likely to necessitate arthroscopic release [45].

Trans-rotator cuff portals can lead to iatrogenic tears, pain, or weakness if not properly placed. In a review of 6 patients with rotator cuff tears related to trans-cuff SLAP repairs, Stephenson emphasizes the need to place these portals medially through the rotator cuff muscle or myotendinous junction [47]. The authors highlight use of a spinal needle as an appropriate tool to localize the proper angle of insertion while staying medial to the rotator cuff tendons. When this is done properly, good outcomes can be obtained when repairing SLAP lesions through trans-rotator cuff portals [47].

Injury to the suprascapular nerve as a result of anchor perforation through the glenoid neck is another iatrogenic complication that has been recently reported in the literature. Numerous anatomic studies have highlighted the danger to the suprascapular nerve that exists during anchor placement due to the close proximity of the nerve to the glenoid neck. Shishido et al. showed that the suprascapular nerve is an average of 2.3 cm from the glenoid rim at the level of the suprascapular notch, and 1.4 cm from the rim at the base of the scapular spine [48]. Cadaveric studies have provided conflicting data over rates of anchor perforation and nerve injury. Anterior anchor perforation rates range from 29 to 100 % when placed through an anterosuperior portal with anchors touching the suprascapular nerve anywhere from 8 to 33 % of the time [49, 50]. Anchor perforation has also been reported for posterior anchors (11 o'clock position) and far posterior anchors (9 o'clock position) through anterior, posterior, portal of Wilmington, and rotator interval portals in varying reports [49, 50]. Further study is necessary to elucidate the safest portal for anchor placement during SLAP repair to minimize the risk of medial glenoid perforation and suprascapular nerve injury.

9.9   Summary

Since the initial recognition of injury patterns specific to the superior labrum/
biceps tendon complex nearly 30 years ago, our understanding of the SLAP lesion
continues to grow. Much research has gone into understanding the relevant
anatomy, biomechanics, pathophysiology, clinical presentation, diagnosis and
treatment of these injuries. Despite this, conflicting data and a lack of level I and II
outcomes data leaves many questions unanswered and many topics in this area
controversial.

So what can we conclude based on the available evidence, in 2013, about the
diagnosis, evaluation and management of SLAP tears?

- The superior labrum/biceps tendon complex is a loose, mobile interface with
  variable attachments to the glenoid. Recognition of these common anatomic
  variants is crucial to proper diagnosis and treatment. Repair of sublabral
  foramen, recesses or other "normal" variants is unnecessary and may be of
  detriment to the patient.
- The diagnosis of SLAP tears remains a difficult task and must be based on a
  combination of the appropriate data gleaned from the clinical history, presenting symptoms, physical exam and imaging studies. There remains no single
  provocative test to isolate SLAP lesions, however, the concept of "the suspicious exam" proposed by Burns and Synder [4] is a useful step in the diagnostic
  algorithm.
- MR arthrography is the standard in imaging for diagnosing SLAP tears, while
  arthroscopic evaluation remains the gold standard in diagnosis.
- For all patients with or without a confirmed diagnosis, initial non-operative
  management with a rehabilitation course focused on scapular stabilization and
  RTC strengthening should be employed, as this may be successful in up to
  70 % of patients. Only after failed conservative treatment should surgery be
  considered.
- Surgical management remains controversial and is dependent on multiple
  factors including the type of SLAP tear, age of the patient, activity level, and
  whether or not the patient participates in overhead throwing sports. Though not
  conclusive, current evidence is more and more suggestive of better results for
  biceps tenodesis and debridement in patients over age 40, especially those with
  biceps tendon damage and/or concomitant rotator cuff tears.
- For type II SLAP repairs, no biomechanical or clinical data exists to suggest
  that a certain suture anchor configuration or suture type provides better results.
  Data does support use of suture anchors over bioabsorbable tacks.
- Long term outcomes data suggest that excellent outcome results and return to
  play can be expected for type II SLAP repairs. There is some conflict over
  whether or not this holds true for patients over 40. Patients receiving worker's
  compensation, and those participating in overhead sports, especially throwers
  consistently have less robust outcomes and return to pre-injury activity level.

- Patients undergoing revision procedures have lower functional scores and patient satisfaction
- Complication incidence is 4.4 % and SLAP repair is not a benign procedure. Stiffness, iatrogenic rotator cuff tear, and suprascapular nerve injury are well recognized, manageable, and potentially avoidable issues.
- More prospective, randomized controlled trials are necessary to delineate better diagnostic criteria, normal anatomic variants versus age related degenerative changes, advantageous repair configurations, rehabilitation protocols, repair versus tenodesis based on age and/or activity level, and ways to minimize iatrogenic complications.

Current evidence has provided a solid framework for the diagnosis and management of SLAP tears. Areas of controversy and conflicting data emphasize the need for focused, well-designed research to answer remaining questions. The popularity of this topic is highlighted by the increasing incidence of SLAP repair, however, care must be taken not to over-diagnose or treat this relatively uncommon injury. Stronger, conclusive research will help identify the patient-specific, evidence based indications for proper treatment of SLAP tears in the future.

References:

1. Andrews JR, Carson WG Jr, McLeod WD (1985) Glenoid labrum tears related to the long head of the biceps. Am J Sports Med 13(5):337
2. Snyder SJ, Karzel RP, Del Pizzo W, Ferkel RD, Friedman MJ (1990) SLAP lesions of the shoulder. Arthrosc: J Arthrosc Relat Surg (Official publication of the Arthroscopy Association of North America and the International Arthroscopy Association) 6(4):274
3. Snyder SJ, Banas MP, Karzel RP (1995) An analysis of 140 injuries to the superior glenoid labrum. J Shoulder Elbow Surg (American Shoulder and Elbow Surgeons [et al]) 4(4):243
4. Burns JP, Bahk M, Snyder SJ (2011) Superior labral tears: repair versus biceps tenodesis. J Shoulder Elbow Surg (American Shoulder and Elbow Surgeons [et al]) 20(2 Suppl):S2
5. Boileau P, Parratte S, Chuinard C, Roussanne Y, Shia D, Bicknell R (2009) Arthroscopic treatment of isolated type II SLAP lesions: biceps tenodesis as an alternative to reinsertion. Am J Sports Med 37(5):929
6. Zhang AL, Kreulen C, Ngo SS, Hame SL, Wang JC, Gamradt SC (2012) Demographic trends in arthroscopic SLAP repair in the United States. Am J Sports Med 40(5):1144
7. Weber SC, Martin DF, Seiler JG 3rd, Harrast JJ (2012) Superior labrum anterior and posterior lesions of the shoulder: incidence rates, complications, and outcomes as reported by American board of orthopedic surgery part II candidates. Am J Sports Med 40(7):1538
8. Gorantla K, Gill C, Wright RW (2010) The outcome of type II SLAP repair: a systematic review. Arthrosc: J Arthrosc Relat Surg (Official publication of the Arthroscopy Association of North America and the International Arthroscopy Association) 26(4):537
9. Bain GI, Galley IJ, Singh C, Carter C, Eng K (2012) Anatomic study of the superior glenoid labrum. Clin Anat 26(3):367–376. doi 10.1002/ca.22145. Epub 2012 Sep 21
10. Vangsness CT Jr., Jorgenson SS, Watson T, Johnson DL (1994) The origin of the long head of the biceps from the scapula and glenoid labrum. An anatomical study of 100 shoulders. J Bone Joint Surg Br 76(6):951
11. Davidson PA, Rivenburgh DW (2004) Mobile superior glenoid labrum: a normal variant or pathologic condition? Am J Sports Med 32(4):962

12. Prodromos CC, Ferry JA, Schiller AL, Zarins B (1990) Histological studies of the glenoid labrum from fetal life to old age. J Bone Joint Surg Am 72(9):1344

13. Smith DK, Chopp TM, Aufdemorte TB, Witkowski EG, Jones RC (1996) Sublabral recess of the superior glenoid labrum: study of cadavers with conventional nonenhanced MR imaging, MR arthrography, anatomic dissection, and limited histologic examination. Radiology 201(1):251

14. Waldt S, Metz S, Burkart A, Mueller D, Bruegel M, Rummeny EJ, Woertler K (2006) Variants of the superior labrum and labro-bicipital complex: a comparative study of shoulder specimens using MR arthrography, multi-slice CT arthrography and anatomical dissection. Eur Radiol 16(2):451

15. Sweitzer BA, Thigpen CA, Shanley E, Stranges G, Wienke JR, Storey T, Noonan TJ, Hawkins RJ, Wyland DJ (2012) A comparison of glenoid morphology and glenohumeral range of motion between professional baseball pitchers with and without a history of SLAP repair. Arthrosc: J Arthrosc Relat Surg (Official publication of the Arthroscopy Association of North America and the International Arthroscopy Association) 28(9):1206

16. Forsythe B, Guss D, Anthony SG, Martin SD (2010) Concomitant arthroscopic SLAP and rotator cuff repair. J Bone Joint Surg Am 92(6):1362

17. Maffet MW, Gartsman GM, Moseley B (1995) Superior labrum-biceps tendon complex lesions of the shoulder. Am J Sports Med 23(1):93

18. Gobezie R, Zurakowski D, Lavery K, Millett PJ, Cole BJ, Warner JJ (2008) Analysis of interobserver and intraobserver variability in the diagnosis and treatment of SLAP tears using the Snyder classification. Am J Sports Med 36(7):1373

19. Mileski RA, Snyder SJ (1998) Superior labral lesions in the shoulder: pathoanatomy and surgical management. J Am Acad Orthop Surg 6(2):121

20. Burkhart SS, Morgan CD (1998) The peel-back mechanism: its role in producing and extending posterior type II SLAP lesions and its effect on SLAP repair rehabilitation. Arthrosc: J Arthrosc Relat Surg (Official publication of the Arthroscopy Association of North America and the International Arthroscopy Association) 14(6):637

21. Hegedus EJ, Goode AP, Cook CE, Michener L, Myer CA, Myer DM, Wright AA (2012) Which physical examination tests provide clinicians with the most value when examining the shoulder? Update of a systematic review with meta-analysis of individual tests. Br J Sports Med 46(14):964

22. Calvert E, Chambers GK, Regan W, Hawkins RH, Leith JM (2009) Special physical examination tests for superior labrum anterior posterior shoulder tears are clinically limited and invalid: a diagnostic systematic review. J Clin Epidemiol 62(5):558

23. Cook C, Beaty S, Kissenberth MJ, Siffri P, Pill SG, Hawkins RJ (2012) Diagnostic accuracy of five orthopedic clinical tests for diagnosis of superior labrum anterior posterior (SLAP) lesions. J Shoulder Elbow Surg (American Shoulder and Elbow Surgeons [et al]) 21(1):13

24. Cook C (2012) Diagnostic accuracy of tests and measures for shoulder labral dysfunction. J Shoulder Elbow Surg 21(11):e20

25. O'Driscoll SW (2012) Regarding "diagnostic accuracy of five orthopedic clinical tests for diagnosis of superior labrum anterior posterior (SLAP) lesions". J Shoulder Elbow Surg 21(12):e23–24. doi: 10.1016/j.jse.2012.08.006. Epub 2012 Oct 26

26. Kibler WB, Sciascia A, Hester P, Jacobs C (2012) Regarding "Diagnostic accuracy of five orthopedic clinical tests for diagnosis of superior labrum anterior posterior (SLAP) lesions". J Shoulder Elbow Surg (American Shoulder and Elbow Surgeons [et al]) 21(9):e16

27. Phillips JC, Cook C, Beaty S, Kissenberth MJ, Siffri P, Hawkins RJ (2012) Validity of noncontrast magnetic resonance imaging in diagnosing superior labrum anterior-posterior tears. J Shoulder Elbow Surg 22(1):3–8. doi: 10.1016/j.jse.2012.03.013. Epub 2012 Aug 29

28. Amin MF, Youssef AO (2012) The diagnostic value of magnetic resonance arthrography of the shoulder in detection and grading of SLAP lesions: comparison with arthroscopic findings. Eur J Radiol 81(9):2343

29. Edwards SL, Lee JA, Bell JE, Packer JD, Ahmad CS, Levine WN, Bigliani LU, Blaine TA (2010) Nonoperative treatment of superior labrum anterior posterior tears: improvements in pain, function, and quality of life. Am J Sports Med 38(7):1456

30. Keener JD, Brophy RH (2009) Superior labral tears of the shoulder: pathogenesis, evaluation, and treatment. J Am Acad Orthop Surg 17(10):627

31. Domb BG, Ehteshami JR, Shindle MK et al (2007) Biomechanical comparison of 3 suture anchor configurations for repair of type II SLAP lesions. Arthroscopy 23:135

32. Yoo JC, Ahn JH, Lee SH et al (2008) A biomechanical comparison of repair techniques in posterior type II superior labral anterior and posterior (SLAP) lesions. J Shoulder Elbow Surg 17:144

33. Boddula MR, Adamson GJ, Gupta A, McGarry MH, Lee TQ (2012) Restoration of labral anatomy and biomechanics after superior labral anterior-posterior repair: comparison of mattress versus simple technique. Am J Sports Med 40(4):875

34. Neri BR, ElAttrache NS, Owsley KC, Mohr K, Yocum LA (2011) Outcome of type II superior labral anterior posterior repairs in elite overhead athletes: Effect of concomitant partial-thickness rotator cuff tears. Am J Sports Med 39(1):114

35. Kim SJ, Lee IS, Kim SH, Woo CM, Chun YM (2012) Arthroscopic repair of concomitant type II SLAP lesions in large to massive rotator cuff tears: comparison with Biceps tenotomy. Am J Sports Med 40(12):2786–2793

36. Abbot AE, Li X, Busconi BD (2009) Arthroscopic treatment of concomitant superior labral anterior posterior (SLAP) lesions and rotator cuff tears in patients over the age of 45 years. Am J Sports Med 37(7):1358

37. Franceschi F, Longo UG, Ruzzini L, Rizzello G, Maffulli N, Denaro V (2008) No advantages in repairing a type II superior labrum anterior and posterior (SLAP) lesion when associated with rotator cuff repair in patients over age 50: a randomized controlled trial. Am J Sports Med 36(2):247

38. Denard PJ, Ladermann A, Burkhart SS (2012) Long-term outcome after arthroscopic repair of type II SLAP lesions: results according to age and workers' compensation status. Arthrosc: J Arthrosc Relat Surg (Official publication of the Arthroscopy Association of North America and the International Arthroscopy Association) 28(4):451

39. Schroder CP, Skare O, Gjengedal E, Uppheim G, Reikeras O, Brox JI (2012) Long-term results after SLAP repair: A 5-Year follow-up study of 107 patients with comparison of patients aged over and under 40 Years. Arthrosc: J Arthrosc Relat Surg (Official publication of the Arthroscopy Association of North America and the International Arthroscopy Association) 28(11):1601

40. Kanatli U, Ozturk BY, Bolukbasi S (2011) Arthroscopic repair of type II superior labrum anterior posterior (SLAP) lesions in patients over the age of 45 years: a prospective study. Arch Orthop Trauma Surg 131(8):1107

41. Sayde WM, Cohen SB, Ciccotti MG, Dodson CC (2012) Return to play after Type II superior labral anterior-posterior lesion repairs in athletes: a systematic review. Clin Orthop Relat Res 470(6):1595

42. Neuman BJ, Boisvert CB, Reiter B, Lawson K, Ciccotti MG, Cohen SB (2011) Results of arthroscopic repair of type II superior labral anterior posterior lesions in overhead athletes: assessment of return to preinjury playing level and satisfaction. Am J Sports Med 39(9):1883

43. Brockmeier SF, Voos JE, Williams RJ 3rd, Altchek DW, Cordasco FA, Allen AA (2009) Outcomes after arthroscopic repair of type-II SLAP lesions. J Bone Joint Surg Am 91(7):1595

44. Park S, Glousman RE (2011) Outcomes of revision arthroscopic type II superior labral anterior posterior repairs. Am J Sports Med 39(6):1290

45. Weber SC (2010) Surgical management of the failed SLAP repair. Sports Med Arthrosc Rev 18(3):162

46. Katz LM, Hsu S, Miller SL, Richmond JC, Khetia E, Kohli N, Curtis AS (2009) Poor outcomes after SLAP repair: descriptive analysis and prognosis. Arthrosc: J Arthrosc Relat

Surg (Official publication of the Arthroscopy Association of North America and the International Arthroscopy Association) 25(8):849

47. Stephenson DR, Hurt JH, Mair SD (2012) Rotator cuff injury as a complication of portal placement for superior labrum anterior-posterior repair. J Shoulder Elbow Surg (American Shoulder and Elbow Surgeons [et al]) 21(10):1316

48. Shishido H, Kikuchi S (2001) Injury of the suprascapular nerve in shoulder surgery: an anatomic study. J Shoulder Elbow Surg 10:372–6

49. Koh HK, Park WH, Lim TK, Yoo JC (2011) Medial perforation of the glenoid neck following SLAP repair places the suprascapular nerve at risk: a cadaveric study. J Shoulder Elbow Surg 20:245–250

50. Chan H, Beaupre LA, Bouliane MJ (2010) Injury of the suprascapular nerve during arthroscopic repair of labral tears: an anatomic study. J Shoulder Elbow Surg 19:709–715

GPSR Compliance

The European Union's (EU) General Product Safety Regulation (GPSR) is a set of rules that requires consumer products to be safe and our obligations to ensure this.

If you have any concerns about our products, you can contact us on ProductSafety@springernature.com

In case Publisher is established outside the EU, the EU authorized representative is:

Springer Nature Customer Service Center GmbH
Europaplatz 3
69115 Heidelberg, Germany

Batch number: 09636590

Printed by Printforce, the Netherlands